Move it to Lose it

Move it to Lose it

CAROL DEXTER

TATE PUBLISHING
AND **ENTERPRISES**, LLC

Published by Tate Publishing & Enterprises, LLC
127 E. Trade Center Terrace | Mustang, Oklahoma 73064 USA
1.888.361.9473 | www.tatepublishing.com

Tate Publishing is committed to excellence in the publishing industry. The company reflects the philosophy established by the founders, based on Psalm 68:11,
"The Lord gave the word and great was the company of those who published it."

Book design copyright © 2014 by Tate Publishing, LLC. All rights reserved.
Cover design by Jim Villaflores
Interior design by Mary Jean Archival

Published in the United States of America

ISBN: 978-1-63063-138-3
1. Health & Fitness / General
2. Health & Fitness / Diet & Nutrition / Weight Loss
14.01.13

Dedications

I would like to dedicate this book to the readers who want to get motivated, to start moving just a little bit more for health and fitness sake.

I do wish to dedicate this book to my brother, Jim, who is as committed to exercise as I am. Jim is always an inspiration to me.

I finally wish to dedicate this book to my many friends, who believed in me to follow through with my dream. Thank you.

Acknowledgements

I wish to personally thank Erin Guidry for his hours of help and expertise in putting this book in manuscript format from the start. I could not have done this on my own.

I also want to thank Susan Guidry, Erin's mother for her unwavering offer of help.

I want to thank Erika, Lori, Susan, and Maria for their constant support and encouragement while at transformations.

I do thank the staff at Tate Publishing for making this book a reality.

Contents

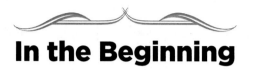

In the Beginning

On my way to dairy queen for my treat of the week—a Cookies and Cream blizzard, I might add—I decided to write this book. I know I shouldn't have had a dairy queen blizzard, but after you read this book, you will know in time that you too will be able to lose weight, enjoy exercise, look great, and eat dessert once in a while (or fairly frequently) should you desire.

All diet and nutrition experts in the world stress the importance of eating the right food for your body, as I do. I am, by no means, an expert in nutrition. However, having taken countless classes and studied nutrition for over thirty years, especially as it pertains to health and weight loss, I do know a fair amount about the subject. Besides, there are so many different opinions out there, and even among the experts I believe one has to do what is best for his or her body by staying within the boundaries of good health. I also believe that instead of always munching on carrots and celery when you get the urge to have a snack, you ought to live a little once in a while and satisfy that urge. The key, however, is to get right back on track. I'll show you how you can eat treats and still reach that goal weight that you've always fantasized about and let you see that all it takes is for you to actually look forward to each new day simply by changing your eating habits ever so slightly in many cases and moving your body.

Years ago when I was still a nursing student, I worked in the cafeteria on weekends to help cover my expenses. Having come from a strict Christian upbringing that forbids snacking between meals (and having to eat everything on my plate at the meals because we were always told that people were starving in India and China, so we were not to waste food whether we liked it or not), I couldn't believe the abundance of food in a cafeteria! No one was there to tell me about the starving people in China, or how bad too much sugar was for my teeth. I was in food heaven! As a result, I went through training pigging out most of the time. Off hours, I would go to the midnight cafeteria in the so-called "dungeon" below the hospital and load up on anything sweet, and before you knew it, I gained thirty pounds. I went from 118 pounds to 114, but for what it's worth, I thought I still looked good—big breasts, fairly small waist, small hips, a rounded belly (but Marilyn Monroe-rounded type of bellies were only in those days, right?) What did I know, the boys were still constantly coming around.

My close friends and I would often fast throughout the week and literally binge for the entire weekend, and little did we know then what havoc starving and binging played on our metabolic rate. I, being the ring leader, tried to *outfast* the others for a whole week, and at the end of a particular week, as we were getting ready to go out, I passed out in the shower from not eating for the week. I hit my head so hard on the tile floor I ended up in the hospital with a concussion. When I got back to my dorm room the next night, I felt so sorry for myself that all I could think about was eating something really gooey. So I did, but then I felt even more miserable. On top of everything else, I ended up gaining a few pounds after fasting all week. How foolish we are when we feel sorry for ourselves. No one puts us in that place but ourselves, yet sometimes it is as though we can't help ourselves and we do it again and again.

One day, someone took a candid photo of me in my student nurse's uniform, and that was all it took to start the diet yo-yo for the next twenty-two years of my life. It's amazing how our emotions and mood dictate our eating habits. It seems we either binge or starve when we are frustrated. Unfortunately, as women, most tend to overeat, and this isn't just a female phenomenon. Men also tend to get a little moodier than women do, in case you haven't noticed. In fact, I think it would be great fun to hide a camera in a car to see how a man reacts to stress when he's alone. I'd bet he snacks more than he would ever admit. Gentlemen, I do say this in general. Please don't take offense.

The best way to lose weight and get into great shape is exercise, and hopefully as you read this book, that message will be made loud and clear. My job here is to help you learn how to enjoy movement of any kind whether you are overweight or just want to maintain your weight. You may not have a reason, and perhaps you are like me— someone who would simply like to be a body in motion.

So please sit back, enjoy, and move it to lose it.

"I believe the good Lord gave us a finite number of heartbeats and I'll be darned if I'm going to use any of mine running up and down a street."—Neil Armstrong

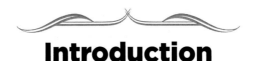

Introduction

Generally speaking, *Move It to Lose It* is a light-hearted book about learning to enjoy exercise—that is, if you haven't yet. I tend to be humorous in life, at work, and at play, and I write that way. I personally feel laughter is a great neutralizer. Years ago, I was in high-end fine arts sales. There were thirty of us salespeople, and the owner stood in front of us and said, "Listen to Carol. She'll talk someone into a ten thousand-dollar painting, and they'll still be laughing as they hand over their credit card." I don't do it to make fun of others by any means; it just seems to be part of my nature to get people to smile, at least.

In spite of the hundreds of diet and exercise books in the marketplace, 60% of the population is still overweight. About 40% don't ever exercise, and 25% exercise so occasionally it hardly counts. It is like what the TV AD says: A body at rest stays at rest, while a body in motion stays in motion. That is a fact. I didn't make that up!

I want people to enjoy reading this book, to at least smile and say to yourself, "I can do that!" I've had many crazy experiences that I'm particularly not proud of, but

I did them and have to take blame for them in the name of binging. Hopefully, many of you will be able to realize you aren't alone out there.

Even though this book is primarily about exercise, I've also talked a bit about nutrition, particularly pertaining to weight loss since the two go hand in hand. I don't claim to be an expert. I'm not. I had two years of training as a nurse then dropped out and put myself through college, working as a nurse in a doctor's office for four and a half years until I got my bachelor's degree in languages and with a minor in biology. After graduating, I was in medical sales for four years and had to train in New Jersey where we were given very intensive training in pharmacology and nutrition as it pertains to drugs and side effects of those drugs.

Later, I continued on my own studying kinesiology, fitness, and nutrition again, since that's the field I wanted to be in over the years, along with my other passion—fine arts! For years now, I've been working as a weight loss consultant, with a sideline in personal training, exercise, and motivational speaking about fitness.

The chapters of this book are short and easy to read. The end of each chapter has a funny quote by a known personality who has been recognized.

I wish you an enjoyable read.

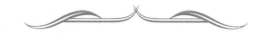

30 Minutes a Day Will Add 10 Years to Your Life

I once knew a very funny man; he was the life of the party and always made fun of me because I'd rather put on jogging shoes than high heels. After work, they'd all go to a bar for a few drinks for happy hour, while I would go jog. He used to say, "Carol, all that exercise has got to be sooo boring! Stop and enjoy life. Life should be one big party because you might die tomorrow." Unfortunately, he treated life like that—he made a great living, worked hard, played harder, drank heavily, ate high fat meals, loved to eat out, gave lavish parties, and absolutely hated exercise. He used to say he swam a lot and that it was exercise enough for him, but swimming for him was getting into water, getting completely wet, paddling around for ten seconds, then getting out. I'm sorry to say though that at the age of forty-nine, he died of a massive heart attack, leaving behind an ex wife and three children.

I can tell you story after story like that, but this book is to motivate you and make you feel good about wanting to start moving, so enough sad stories!

On a daily basis, I talk to people who seem utterly shocked that in order to lose weight and get into shape they absolutely have to change their eating habits and start moving their bodies not just at work. I honestly think many people—mostly men—feel that there must be a little magic fairy that sprinkles fairy dust over them and the excess fat will automatically go away and their bodies will become buff and beautiful again. If that were the case, weight loss clinics would be the most lucrative businesses in the world. Nothing is easy. People had a great time putting all that extra weight on, but when it comes to taking it off, it does take work and discipline. It can be done though, and I guarantee it with every fiber of my being.

Here are some more great tips to make an exercise a small part of your day: drop the all-or-nothing attitude. Stop saying "I'm going to join a gym" or "I've just joined a gym." Just go to the gym! If it is too difficult to get there, buy a used treadmill and put it in your home, You can always pick one up for fifty dollars. I did and it works great.

Or as I've said countless times before, go for a walk and enjoy the scenery, which leads to another tip: you can save quite a bit on gas by stopping to take your car on every little errand. If you have the extra time, walk to the corner store or cleaners. That is one of the great things you can get when you live in a city. You have to walk everywhere. I would be willing to bet many of your city friends who are used to walking everywhere have very few weight problems.

Years ago, while running several large galleries in San Francisco, since they were only a ½ mile apart and the third was approximately 2 miles further I used to literally walk to all locations instead of driving. I had a car, but the parking in the city was a nightmare and an overwhelming cost, so I often preferred the walk instead, especially when I had the extra time. In the warmer weather, it was magic. For those of you who have been blessed to have spent some time in San Francisco, it is one of the most unique cities in the country and a difficult city to walk in, since there are so many steep hills. To say it kept me extremely fit is putting it mildly. Walking alone makes a huge difference on the scale and, consequently, on your health.

On the other hand, if you work or live in the suburbs or in a semi-rural area—perhaps a stay-home mom, a writer, or someone who just needs to get out for a few minutes—you'll find that being outside in nature renews and lifts your spirits. It gives you a sense of well-being and may act as a calming agent without a tranquilizer. You'll feel like going back in and tackling whatever project or problem that awaits you.

Take every opportunity to move, and I mean that emphatically. Stop worrying what everyone else might think about you or how silly you might look to them. Do you think I care that people teased me over the years why I chose to walk while they go on and drive for a few errands, even at short distances? Or that I preferred to walk around looking at Christmas decorations in spite of the cold while they wanted to drive? Or that I usually stayed for another hour and a half at the gym while they worked out for just thirty minutes? How could I, when now, years later, they all say, "Carol, how I wish I had your figure," or now that they are forty pounds overweight they say they're too tired to exercise? Try carrying around two twenty-pound bags of kitty litter and see if you can. You can't. It's next to impossible. So what's it going to take to get people to see the light? I hope they get on the "move it to lose it" momentum before it becomes too late.

I may have said it before and if I did, I'm sorry but it needs to be said again and again, Exercise is a gift, and you should enjoy the fact that you have two legs that can still move, knees that can bend, arms that can lift, among others. Enjoy something as simple as lifting your small child or grandchild over and over and you'll see how they love to laugh at such a movement. Get on the floor and play piggyback with them. If there are no children around, get on the floor anyway and start doing some abdominal crunches or leg stretches. There are so many simple exercises to get you moving. Personally, I like to do a few basic ones before I start brisk walking or jogging. If I'm playing tennis, on the other hand, I stretch for a few seconds then do a few exercises after I finish playing.

Sometimes in life, we have to step outside our comfort zone. Yours perhaps would be getting up two hours early before you go to work so that you can sit and relax for an hour with your coffee, read the paper, and then leisurely get ready for work. In fact, I had one particular client who had the hardest time losing weight because she simply refused to take the time to exercise, even for just an hour every other day. When she told me she needed this early time for herself, I said, "Well, you also want to lose that extra thirty pounds. Don't you think that would be an exceptional goal? And isn't it worth sacrificing at least half of your early coffee and paper time to help you attain that weight loss by simply walking for a half hour each day?" She very reluctantly agreed, but at least she took the challenge. Eventually, she finally lost weight. It took her a little longer because she wasn't willing to give up the whole hour, but the point is, she did compromise and it worked!

Whatever you need to do to start moving, just do it, just start moving. Little by little it will pay off. Once you truly commit to doing something beyond your normal daily activities, you will lose the weight. I guarantee it.

> "The trouble with jogging is by the time you realize you are not in shape for it, it is too far to walk back."—Franklin P. Jones

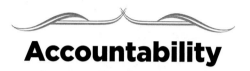

Accountability

I once had a doctor tell me that the best way to tell if you are truly fit is to stand in front of a full-length mirror, naked. I did and I thought, *okay, so far so good. I looked pretty fit for an aging lady.* Then he said, "Turn sideways and bend over from the waist and look in the mirror. If you see any flesh hanging over anywhere, you are not fit."

Needless to say, after doing this little exercise, I was totally demoralized. I thought I was in such great shape and was I ever wrong! The sagging stomach ruled. Like a madwoman, I started doing as many abdominal crunches as I could physically handle and any additional exercise that I thought would cut down the sagging tummy. I was so shocked at how bad I looked in that position that I didn't even want to eat. Unfortunately, that feeling didn't last very long, only for a day or two at the maximum.

This leads me into accountability. True, it is so difficult to stay focused on your own when it comes to losing weight. You feel like you are alone in the world, even though you know there are thousands of other people out there with the same problem. In your immediate group of family and friends, others may say they are going to start a diet soon—typically over a big lunch or dinner—but are they actually doing it? It is a personal issue and one you wouldn't want to talk about. I'm sure you know a few people who always say they are going on a diet, but over the years they still stay the same—forty pounds overweight.

I have a friend who, I think, is one of the most beautiful women I know, but every time I see her (she lived out of state, so we got together once or twice a year), the first thing she'd say year in and year out is "I've just got to go on a diet." Now, thirty years later, she's still saying it. I'm so tired of hearing this that many times I've been tempted to say "Either shut up about your weight or do something about it!" However, I know that would hurt her feelings, so I just keep the thought to myself. It's a shame that often we feel we can't be honest to our friends, who are closest to us, for fear of losing the friendship when in the long run, if we were honest we would be helping them immensely.

Unfortunately, mirrors and scales don't lie. You'd like to believe the doctor's scale at his office had to be wrong because you know you don't weigh that much. But you're wrong. 99.9% of the time, the medical scales are far more accurate than our home scales. We all need support, whether it is in losing weight or starting a new exercise regimen. A friend here at work said she started going to the gym and yet, she doesn't even take the time to go regularly. Like I said, until something becomes a habit, it does take motivation and commitment to stay with the program. That's where weight loss clinics come in. All the employees at the clinics are there not only to teach you to correct your eating habits and lifestyle but also to give you support and encouragement along the way. If it were so easy on your own, then there would be no need for the countless weight loss centers out there, and most likely, our country would have far more obese people with major illnesses.

Usually, we never see ourselves the way others see us, which is one reason why we put off the inevitable. When you try to start a weight loss program on your own, oftentimes you give in to temptations. It is so easy to think you had a bad day so then you would deserve pizza or a cheeseburger, fries, and a shake. I know, I've been there a thousand times in my life and definitely know what it's like when your significant other tells you, "Honey, you still look fine to me," and you don't know whether to hit him or hug him. But simply say, "Thank you, but I'm doing this for me," and privately you may grit your teeth and tell yourself you're going to look not just fine but fabulous. Now that's a motivation.

A company that is very dear to my heart is Transformations Medical Weight Loss They have been around for over twenty-five years and have many locations that are primarily centered in Florida. The minute you walk through their doors, you would feel so welcomed and that you are the most important person in the world. Everyone is just as caring—the receptionist, counselors, nurses, and even doctors. You don't feel like it is about the money with them but that it's primarily about your desire to lose weight, and they are with you every step of the way. Transformations also encourages exercise as well.

There are countless clinics and weight loss centers out there in the marketplace. Some want you to buy their food products, some are very expensive, some give you "cookies," some use only natural products, some use celebrities to get their point across, while others advertise potentially misleading claims. Very rarely does a person lose thirty-plus pounds in a month. Realistically, the average that women lose is approximately twelve pounds a month, while men tend to lose a few more pounds. This, of course, is just an average. Some people lose more, while others lose less. You always have to take into consideration a lot of variables: how overweight a person is in the first place, how active a person is, how committed, how long on the diet, medical conditions, to name a few.

The point is, no matter which weight loss center you go with, the staff is there for you. They all bring something to the table to help you. It just depends on what you feel is the best program for you. Take advantage of them. If it helps you lose the forty pounds you've talked about losing for the last twenty-five years, don't you think it is well worth the price? I do. I can't help but believe we only live once, so be as healthy and in shape as you can be.

> "Oh, that this solid flesh would melt."—William Shakespeare

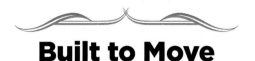

Built to Move

The greatest machine God ever created is the human body. Think of all the moveable parts we have controlled by our internal computer that is our brain. Simply put, an area in our brain sends signals throughout our body that tell our muscles to move, which enable our head, neck, shoulders, arms, hands, hips, knees, legs, feet, and all the tiny parts in between to move. Of course, the most important organ of all is the heart, without which we wouldn't exist. How wonderful the human body is that we don't even have to think about our moveable parts; they just work. And until you have an injury, illness, or surgery, you don't even give them a second thought, but when the day comes that you can't move all those parts, you realize how special it is to just do it!

Recently, after undergoing back surgery, I was not able to lift, bend, or twist for three months. Try going through your normal daily routines without being able to do these things. It was an act of god just to be able to get out of bed without bending. We take for granted simple tasks like putting on pants, tying shoestrings, and brushing our teeth. I couldn't even bend my neck to rinse out my mouth after brushing. To put on my scrubs for work, I had to lie flat on the bed, raise my legs, and pray that I could get each leg in the right opening. I won't even discuss how I tried to go to the bathroom for the first few weeks without bending or twisting!

The point is to be grateful for the ability to move. Having had the brief experience mentioned above makes me have the greatest respect for those who can't move, yet deal with it every day of their lives. There are so many in wheelchairs who would give anything just to be able to walk again, even for just a day, while so many others complain about having to walk a little further away because someone took the parking space they wanted right in front of the store.

Other people can't move due to years of bad eating habits. Approximately 70% of chronic illnesses are caused by what we put in our stomachs. As the years go by, you don't think about the damage you are doing internally. The majority of the restaurants specialize in fried foods. They create ads that make the food look so tantalizing, and as a result, the kids say, "Can we go there, Mom?" Being the sweet mom that you are, you say, "Okay, as soon as your father gets home from work." After dinner, you justify what you ate, even though the chicken was fried, it was still protein. The peas and corn smothered in butter were vegetables, and vegetables are good for us, right? The pie for dessert was apple-flavored, so you had fruit, only it was buried under two scoops of butter pecan ice cream. If this were an occasional event, it wouldn't matter, but in thousands of homes across the US, that's how it usually goes during dinnertime, whether at home or out.

Pizza loaded with cheese, or a meat lovers' version with extra cheese in the crust is another artery-clogging food we all love. If you have to have a pizza night once in a while, avoid loading it with fatty meats. At least, select one lean meat, if available, and I don't mean sausage or bacon, not even turkey bacon. And don't add any more pork products. A lean round, steak, chicken, or shrimp would work very well with 2% cheese, marinara sauce, or a light cream sauce with arugula or broccoli and mushrooms. Or better yet, get a vegetarian pizza. Instead of eating two or three slices, slowly eat one slice. If you absolutely have to have a pepperoni pizza, keep it down to one slice. Pepperoni is another high fat meat that will do you no good other than a heartburn. I would be willing to bet that most children prefer just cheese on their pizza. Cherish that and hope that they will continue to prefer that. Cheese is better.

There are so many other foods that are really harmful in the grand scheme of things. Personally, I absolutely love Chinese food. It doesn't even have to be really good. I can't begin to count how many times I've had Chinese at the mall food courts. All the sweet tangy sauces and heavily-breaded fried coatings they use actually mask the miniscule amount of meat used. In most cases, it is hard to tell. I typically try to order skinless teriyaki chicken or other entrées where I can see the actual meat or fish. Fried rice too is shockingly high in fat content and calories. Since I learned that there is often over 1,200 calories and thirty grams of fat in it, I've learned to make one myself. That way I can control the ingredients.

You may wonder why I'm spending so much time on these, but your eating habits are an integral part of your journey to weight loss. What you eat can cause you to get so sluggish that you don't feel like moving. A lot of foods cause bloating, sleepiness, upset stomach, and headaches, and because you don't feel like moving around, your metabolism drops, and you not only gain weight but your body also stores all the excess as fat, which can lead to serious illnesses and even death. There may be times when you just want something fatty or fried. Eat it then move on. The point is to allow yourself a splurge once in a while. Too many people can't stop with one splurge, and the next day they would do it again. Hopefully, if you aren't accustomed to eating these kinds of food, you will feel so miserable afterward that you eagerly get right back into healthy eating habits for the next meal.

When I eat something that may taste great, I find it always going down but leaving behind such a bad aftertaste or stomach irritation, but not until I get up and walk around a bit. But if you just sit or lie down there in front of the TV, guaranteed, you will feel miserable all night. Again, it is always better to get up and move wherever you are. Just do it. Why should you treat your body, your very personal machine, with so much abuse that most food unfortunately cause? Just like a car, it will dull, thicken, and wear down to the point of not being able to run anymore.

When symptoms such as being tired, run down, sleepy, weak, and having no energy do occur, you tend to blame it on everything else most, if not all, of the time, except on what you eat. You say, "I'm just getting old, or my joints are stiff, or I have bad knees, so I can't walk much." If you try walking a little each day and have one less slice of pizza, or a little less dessert, you will surprise yourself; it does work. You are what you eat, and if you eat right or at least less than what you usually shove in your mouth, you can move more and enjoy it. Ironically, when that happens, you will find that you actually want to eat less of the bad stuff and more of the good stuff.

My father died suddenly at age of sixty-nine. All his life, he worked hard. In those days, it was the husband's place to earn the living to care for his family. The wife's responsibility was to stay at home, raise the family, and maintain the upkeep of the house. In my parents' home, they always made it a point to prepare dinner before five forty-five in the evening. The point is, my father put in nine hours in his shifts every day of his life until he was sixty-five. Each night, he would come home from work, sit down, read the paper if he hadn't read it at work, and then watch TV until dinnertime. He was always so stiff, as though his knees refused to bend every time he tried to get out of the chair. After dinner, he would get up stiff-legged and again sit down in front of the TV until bedtime. This was his life year after year. My father wasn't the kind to go out and play ball with his son or take us hiking in the woods.

When we did do something as a family outside though, it was usually a Sunday afternoon drive. But that was it. We drove, often to visit friends, and when we got to their homes, we would once again sit. That's probably one reason why I've become so addicted to being outside and exercising for hours. I had such a sedentary childhood that I felt like making up for lost time. I look back at those times and think how sad it all was. Perhaps, had he taken better care of himself and got into, at least, nightly walks as his physical exercise, he might still be alive today. You just can't blame stiff joints and arthritis on old age.

You can stay completely mobile and agile even well into your nineties as long as you do some physical activity. A doctor told me years ago that if it weren't for my daily exercise habit, I too could have had severe arthritis. It can start at a young age, but exercise will keep it in check. Think about an old car or a lawn mower. It gets rusty and so rigid that it can't move unless you oil it well or even replace parts and use it from time to time. It is no different from our human machine. You have to move it to use it so that you can lose it!

> "A man's health can be judged by which he takes two at a time—pills or stairs."—Joan Welsh

Call a Friend

Have you ever noticed how much you laugh when you are talking to a close friend, even perhaps, if it's just through a phone call, email, or just lunch or coffee in the morning? We cherish our close friends, male or female, although not always but more often than not. In fact, over the years, our significant others may come and go, but our true friends last through thick and thin as the saying goes, which is why we cherish them so. We can say and do as we wish, but our friends usually love us unconditionally almost as much as our beloved pets do.

I have only a handful of really close friends whom I share my most intimate details with. Usually, we laugh or realize how stupid we are, but a friend will always have your back—always. Isn't it funny how a friend can critique on your hair or your weight, and you won't get upset about it, but when your husband or mate criticizes you on the same thing, you go ballistic. I know, told you I've been there and done that.

So why not exercise with them? That is a great way if you haven't already started to do so. A few years ago, while living in Maui, I had a really close friend, who still is one of my very best friends, even though I no longer live in Maui, and we did this four-mile walk together a few times a week. We got so hooked that we always looked forward to this ritual not just for the exercise but for our gossip and laugh session too. Sometimes, we'd be talking and laughing about something so much that we'd be at the end of our walk before we knew it. That's the joy of working out with a friend. It became a great relaxing therapy session instead of an exercise session.

Try it and then make it a weekly habit. It is a fact that women tend to lose more weight when they exercise with a friend, and that's because, in part, I think we are competitive and we love the challenge of seeing who can lose more—you or your friend. Set a goal or a wager with your friend—or better yet, friends. Perhaps, the loser buys movie tickets. It makes losing weight more fun. An upcoming event is always a great goal, even if you have to make up one—you can always set a girls' night out.

If it is someone you work with who needs to lose some weight and is always talking about it, try to light a fire under that person and suggest walking after work or going to the gym together if the gym is close by. I worked with an incredible lady at a weight loss center a few years ago who always had twenty pounds to lose but could never lose it. When I suggested walking together after work, she always had excuses. When I asked why all the excuses, she said she hated to sweat because it was unfeminine and that she didn't like the sun, the humidity, and the weather condition. I kept on persuading her until she said, "Carol, I guess you won't give up until I walk with you." Eventually, she did, and because she started losing that extra weight she liked walking even more.

You have nothing to lose but weight so remember that! Start moving everyone!

On a brighter note, I know that there's always a part of you that always wants to work up a sweat. That means everything is functioning internally, and your metabolic rate is climbing. So start moving, and remember that in doing so you have nothing to lose but weight.

> "Fitness needs to be perceived as fun and games or we subconsciously avoid it."—Alan Thicke

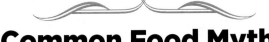

Common Food Myths

1. **You don't have to count calories.** Of course you have to count calories. Too often we "guestimate" how many calories we eat per meal. Usually, we underestimate which is evident by the scale. As a weight loss coach, I figured I would have a dollar every time a client would say to me, "Honest, I really stuck to the diet all week. I don't know why I didn't lose any weight. There must be something wrong with this diet." 99.999% of the time we don't count every calorie we consume. To help you lose weight, I strongly urge you to keep a running diary of every bite and every taste you take. Get a small pocket-size notebook or diary and write down everything as soon as you eat. Don't try to remember every morsel you ate that day before you go to bed at night. Invariably, you'll forget something, either consciously or unconsciously. Statistically, those who keep a daily tally will lose 65% more weight than their counterparts who don't. It helps you become aware of every bite you take so that even on special occasions, you tend to eat less.

2. **Carbs are bad for you; they make you fat.** Why do so many people think this is a fact? We absolutely need carbs to survive. There are, of course, good carbs and bad carbs, simple carbs versus complex carbs. Cake and candy carbs are definitely a no-no. Oatmeal and whole grain carbs, may they be pasta, brown rice, or potatoes, yes. A calorie is a calorie no matter what form it takes. It is a unit of energy your body needs to survive. It's the quantity you take in that gets you into trouble.

3. **You must eat three meals a day.** Ideally one must eat every 3 to 4 hours so that your blood sugar level doesn't crash, giving you that sudden tired feeling. Even a small snack, such as an apple, or a banana, or better yet, a handful of almonds, will help ward off that drop.

4. **You must eat smaller meals four to five times a day.** This too seems to be an ongoing argument, which is why I decided to put them together. Some experts feel it is better for your digestive tract to eat three meals a day with no snacking in between, while others feel you are better off eating a little every few hours then you won't eat so much at your regular meal times. But I say do whatever works the best for you. You know your schedule and what works the best for your body. After all, what matters is the total number of calories you consume each day versus what your body needs. Whenever you eat more than what you need, your body stores it as fat and that's not good for anyone.

5. **Eating late at night is bad for you; it will just make you fat.** It's important to remember that your body has no concept of time. Contrary to some opinions out there of other nutritionists and personal trainers, it doesn't matter when you eat but how much you eat versus what your body needs. If your body, for example, requires 2,000 calories to maintain your weight, and you take in only 1,500 calories, you're bound to slowly lose weight, and no matter what weight loss and exercise program you decide to go with the weight loss, coaches can help you figure out just how many calories you need to maintain your weight.

6. **Just give up everything that has sugar in it and you'll lose weight.** Again, many experts say that sugar is toxic, but I say that if taken moderately, sugar is good, depending too on the conditions of your body. Obviously, if you are diabetic, then it is not good for you. Food is one of life's greatest pleasures to be shared with family and friends. When we interact with others, food is in most cases, if not all, involved. If you eat healthy meals 95% of the time and at some point want to indulge in that birthday cake, which just comes along every once in a while, then go right ahead. That in itself will not hurt you. Eating the whole cake, however, will. I usually justify it by walking an extra few miles when I know I'm going to have dessert, or going to a party, or ten other reasons to indulge. As I've said before, it is always easier to work off sugar than fat calories, so if you have to have a treat, do so with something sweet!

7. **Grapefruit, cabbage, among others, are fat burners.** There are no foods that actually burn fat, just as the myth that sugar makes you fat. Remember the principle, as long as you eat less than what your body needs, you will lose weight and burn fat. This is a far fetched example but years ago and I mean years ago when I went through this "I can eat anything I want and still lose weight phase", I ate only donuts. Yes, that was stupid but I did lose weight because I was eating fewer calories than my body required. You can lose weight on anything when you eat less than what your body needs, end of story. It's a ridiculous unhealthy way to diet, but I did some ridiculous diets in the name of vanity when I was younger. The ideal way to burn fat is to add daily exercise to your diet. If certain foods did burn fat, prices would skyrocket on those items because demand on them would be a constant issue, and farmers would run out of supply.

8. **As long as you exercise, you never have to diet.** That myth has gotten many of us in trouble. For years, I used that excuse to eat all I wanted and anything I wanted. I remember eating out with several men in my past, and they would marvel at how much food I could consume. Every time, I used to say it's because I exercise two hours every day, but I was eating as though I exercised four hours every day! Slowly but surely, I started getting "well-rounded."

One day, a beau said to me, "You are so attractive, Carol, even though you have a belly." That did it. I was so angry that that night I stood in front of a full-length mirror, nude, and was shocked to see how rounded I had become. It's amazing how pounds and fat slowly accumulate, and we just don't want to see ourselves as others see us. Look at yourself naked at a side view, bend over, and see if the image doesn't make you want to move it to lose it. Because you exercise, you make that common mistake of overeating. When you think of how far you have to walk or run to burn off a cheeseburger or a piece of cake, which is approximately eight miles, you are better off not eating it until you are at the weight you want to be.

9. **Protein will never make you fat.** On the contrary, anything, no matter what it is, eaten in excess will make you gain weight. Everything in excess is stored in your body as fat, even protein. Protein can also be harmful when taken in excessive amounts. You have to have healthy kidneys and liver to process high quantities of protein. Also, if you do have a strenuous fitness regimen, your body will require a higher amount of protein; however, you'll also have to increase your water intake. Usually, active females require approximately forty grams of protein daily, but since I do exercise fairly regularly, I take in approximately sixty grams of protein daily.

10. **Like it or not, myths are just that—myths.** The point is, we just have to watch everything we eat to be healthy, happy, and fit.

"The only time to eat diet food is while you're waiting for the steak to cook."—Julia Child

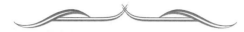

I'm Not Famous, Just Fit

Do you ever notice that all the exercise and fitness ads on television, in magazines, and in newspapers show really fit attractive young men and women? Both have perfectly flat abs, are slender and toned where they need to be toned. The women are also perfectly made up, looking like they are going to a party instead of working out, and the men are muscular with that handsome chiseled look as though they are getting ready for a pinup calendar shoot. The advertising companies would also say: "You too can have perfectly flat abs, toned buttocks and back in just 15 minutes!" But these claims aren't reality and just tend to infuriate me. These ads make this kind of look become the holy grail of fitness and as if it is easy to accomplish.

In the first place, most of mankind are not celebrities, movie stars, and athletes. The majority are ordinary people like you and me, who just want to get into shape and stay in shape. You are not a twenty-something wanna be but someone who wants to look as good as you can with what you've got. So then we ask, why don't these companies ever use real-looking people for their ads?

Because for these people, it is about selling their product and making a profit—a huge profit in most cases. People have to be in business to make money, but I strongly believe there should be an underlying cause and that's to help mankind be healthy and in shape. Average-looking people don't sell, and I think many of us live vicariously through these glamorous people we see on those ads, which is sad because we all are beautiful in our own way.

Years ago, I went out with a man who was indeed average-looking but had such a great personality, and I remember being smitten for years. My friends would always tease me and say, "Honestly, Carol, can't you do any better than that?" The longer I dated this person, the more handsome he became to me. The beauty was internal but in time became external in my eyes, and I'm sure many of you have had that kind of experience. Everyone wants to feel attractive. You may not want to look like a movie star, but you'd probably want to have a flat stomach, and that seems to be the one desire most men and women want in their weight loss aspirations. However, it isn't, in spite of all the ads saying how easy it is to accomplish. The abdominal area is by far the most difficult area to slim down, but the good news is that it can be done. You don't even have to wait until you get a gym membership.

Some of the following steps apply not only to the abs but more importantly to the whole body, which is wonderful because typically, you want to tone everything from head to toe.

1. **Stand up straight.** Improving one's posture is such a simple thing that we rarely do. My friends always nag me about standing up straight, holding shoulders back and the head up high. After years of slouching, the stomach starts to sag, and abs definitely become flabby. Even people with slender frames can develop a sagging abdominal area, yet the minute you stand straight, you automatically pull in that sagging area and look as if you'd instantly lost five pounds. Try doing it while walking at a brisk pace. It will help your whole core group of muscles, back, shoulders, glutes, legs and arms. It actually feels good too. You need to do this every day though, and not just once in a while. That's the key.

2. **Go cycling.** The American council on fitness did a major study a few years ago and found that one of the best ways to tone the abs and core group is to ride a bike, or at the very least, do the imaginary bicycle pump where you are lying on the floor, with your hands behind your head, legs pumping in the air as though you are actually riding a bike. If you don't have a bike, do this exercise for a half hour three times a week, and you will be on your way to an amazingly toned abs, stomach, and legs. Bike riding is not only such a relaxing way to exercise, but it's also a fun way to see sights that you wouldn't be able to see while driving. Try it, and I guarantee you'll love it. Again, the trick is to make it a routine several times a week. Anything

you set out to do as far as getting fit goes has to become a habit. Otherwise, it won't work at all. It's a good thing that all gyms provide stationary bikes for your exercise. The advantage to these equipment in the gyms is that you can increase your speed and intensity whenever you like.

It is amazing that with the advent of technology and all the gimmicks in the marketplace, the good old bike is still one of today's top three best ways to get the firm results you want. The key to any exercise routine is the intensity. For those of you short on time, you can get pretty decent results with only thirty minutes a day. You just have to make that half hour as vigorous and intense as you can handle it to maximize your results. You can do interval work, for instance, ten minutes at a normal speed, average grade, and then go to a hill setting at a little higher speed. This, of course, is if you are at the gym and on a stationary bike. You may do that for ten minutes and then drop the grade and speed again. And if you are doing crunches or lunges, try holding three to five-pound hand weights. Men definitely will have heavier weights, but the point is, whatever it is that you are doing for that thirty-minute period, try to speed up then slow down, speed up again or double up your training with weights. If you are at home and lying flat, hold light weights at arm's length as you do leg raises. This may put a strain on your arms, so do this a few times to start then slowly build.

There certainly are a lot of things you can accomplish in just a thirty-minute exercise session, and despite the many chronic conditions caused by being overweight, anything that you get in the habit of doing for your health's sake is guaranteed to pay off tenfold.

When I went in for my final post op and Xray visit following my back surgery, the surgeon said, "Carol, I don't know what you did to heal so quickly and so well, but your results are beyond belief." He went on to say that my rate of healing was a direct correlation to being fit. And I said, "You told me to walk as much as I could, and I did." Walking not only speeds up recovery from surgery; it also revs up your metabolism, creates a sense of well-being, fights off mood swings, among others. To say that it helps give you lots of energy is putting it mildly. I don't mean just walking around a block or two but pushing yourself a little further each day. Personally, even after a five-mile walk, I felt as though I could walk more, so I did. I often walked early in the day, and then late in the afternoon I'd do it again. I realized it's pretty hard to sit around once your body is in tune with an exercise routine. You feel like you just want to move it.

Once you are comfortable with a routine, no matter what form of physical movement it takes, you'll notice a big difference between feeling drained and revved up. As you start a new program, you'll probably complain about being tired and not having enough energy to continue, and that's when you can't give up, you must continue for a few minutes beyond that feeling. The revved-up stage kicks in and you've won, and you will no longer have that too-tired-to-start-today feeling.

Where ever you are, whenever you feel yourself nodding off, (I used to feel that when I'd be at all day seminars where you literally had to sit still for 6 to 8 hours at a time), I think back to those corporate sales training days and wonder why the corporate execs didn't give us 10 minute walk breaks instead of pastry and coffee breaks. How much better we all would have done! None the less, should you be somewhere and you do feel like nodding off, try to excuse yourself and say you have to make an emergency phone call, if necessary,and go for a brisk 10 minute walk, or go into the restroom and jump up and down or run in place for a few minutes. This will do wonders for your ability to stay alert during those long dragged out meetings. When you suddenly feel overcome with fatigue or sleepiness, have a piece of chocolate, preferably dark chocolate. Better yet, have a dark chocolate-covered mint or two. Mint and dark chocolate is a great pick-me-up. The few extra calories aren't going to sabotage your diet (unless you are eating milk chocolate that's layered over caramel). That's not going to work.

If you have to break down your exercise in 5 or 10 minute intervals whenever you get the chance rather than a one hour break which lends itself to excuses for another day, I suggest you do the 5 minute one 5 or 6 times a day and it will still be as effective as one long session. Make time no matter what. Any time is absolutely better than saying "I have no time to exercise!" I refuse to buy into that and you should too. To look good and feel good, you certainly have to move it!

Craigslist and resale stores often have used exercise equipment such as stationary bikes and treadmills for sale at just a fraction of what you'd pay for new ones. I even buy regular bicycles there because they are so inexpensive that

I don't worry if they get stolen. Not that I want a bike to get stolen, but with the popularity of cycling nowadays, it does happen frequently. Craigslist and other resale stores are a great place to start without breaking the bank. I like to keep a treadmill or recumbent bike at home because it is a constant reminder of working out, even if it's just for a few minutes before your husband comes home or before you have to pick up the kids from school.

There are many excellent natural products on the market that help energize you so that you don't feel too tired to work out. Green tea is an excellent energizer as well as an antioxidant to help fight off the radicals caused by fatty foods in the first place. The amino acid group, especially choline, inositol, L-carnitine, leucine and most other amino acids, is another fantastic source, Basically, they help in fat metabolism and in the redistribution of body fat as well as a multitude of other things. These actions, in turn, help lower cholesterol levels in the body.

Again, do whatever it takes, except overeating, to build up your energy level until your body is conditioned to do it on its own. This happens only when a routine becomes a habit and when it does, you'll never again say, "I'm too tired."

"The only valid excuse for not exercising is paralysis."
—Author: Moira Nordholt, feelgood guru.com

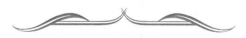

Comfort Food in a Competitive Society

A few years ago, while working in an art gallery in Lahaina, Maui, a young middle-aged woman came in with her mother. I attempted to engage in a conversation with them, but to no avail. Both ignored me and kept chatting about the arts to each other. The daughter, extremely obese, was around thirty-four years old, while the mother, very pretty in a sophisticated way, seemed to be fifty-eight years of age. With the way they acknowledged me—the mother examining me from head to toe in the way that stuffy people have a tendency of doing, and the daughter shyly smiling and saying hello—I could see that to get their attention, I would have to say something fairly witty, which I normally do to break the ice, so to speak. In sales, we are taught to mimic the personality of the person we are speaking to, but sometimes I find that humor works very well. So within a half hour, I had won them over.

I could feel the pain in the daughter's demeanor, but as I questioned them about their interest in this particular artist whose work they were admiring, the daughter immediately became animated. She really loved the work, but the mother quickly put her down,. as if making her feel as though she didn't know good art if it hit her wasn't enough. The daughter was so embarrassed and said, "I'm sorry, Mother, but I do like his art." The mother spoke up then and said, "Fine, you can buy it with your money. You are always spending money frivolously anyway. You wanted to go to chef's school and look what happened, you became fatter than you already were."

Needless to say, the daughter did not buy any work by the artist. The daughter was so ashamed she just meekly left. I felt bad about not making the sale, but more importantly it made me realize how much pain so many people go through in their private worlds. I'm not talking about the physical pain but the mental, which can be far more devastating than the physical. Often you can fix the physical just as easily with surgery or medication, but the mental can take years to undo.

So as all fitness fanatics do, I say just do it. Do it without thinking of how difficult it is for hundreds of thousands of obese people to do. Perhaps growing up in a wealthy environment as this particular woman did was painful because she never felt capable of making her own decisions, and her mother probably always told her she must not over eat or she'd get fat. Her mother might have constantly nagged her about everything that as a result, this shy, plain girl turned into a withdrawn, obese woman who no longer feels good about herself. She then turns to food again and again because it has become her friend, and it made her feel really good.

Years ago, when I was just newly married to a very fit, controlling husband, my husband was so obsessed about fitness that he insisted I stay on a regimented diet to the max. Our meals consisted of fruits, cottage cheese, tuna and other fish, and soft boiled eggs for breakfast every day except for Sundays. I was fortunate for two years anyway because he didn't want me to work. He wanted me to become an outstanding tennis player primarily, a housewife as a secondary role, and as fit and shapely as I could possibly be.

One day while he was at work, I was fantasizing about warm, soft chocolate chip cookies. After three hours of tennis, I drove about thirty miles to a shopping center so that my husband wouldn't know anything about it, and I couldn't wait to buy some mouth-watering cookies just out of the oven. I no sooner bought a half dozen freshly baked cookies and was stuffing one into my mouth as fast as I could when I felt a hand on my shoulder. It was my husband, and he turned to me and said, "Darling, you shouldn't eat that." I was too stunned to speak. He said he was out on an errand and saw me drive by and decided to follow me.

Later that night, I cried because I realized I had no control over what I could and couldn't eat with him in my life. It also gave me a foreboding feeling of what my marriage was going to be like. After all, I had only known him for a month before I married him. I thought I loved this much older, sophisticated, controlling man, so I gave in trying to please him. Now I look back on it and realize how stupid I was, but when you are caught up in an emotional event you do make stupid mistakes. The trick is to grow out of them, learn from them, and move on. There are many situations out there, even today where we allow others to control our eating habits for the sake of love. And worse yet, we use food as a comfort to us because we don't feel "worthy" of another's feelings.

Often, you hear people say (usually family members as indicated before), "honestly, you have to do something about your weight." "You're getting fatter and fatter all the time." Try to put yourself in that person's shoes. You might say they deserve it because they bring it on themselves. But unless you've never had an eating problem you wouldn't know how challenging that is. You have absolutely no idea how miserable people can feel because of their weight. Yet they continue on this downward spiral because they feel less and less about themselves and the only thing that doesn't hurt,is, food Just remember how difficult it is to lose 15 or 20 pounds, so you can imagine what a commitment it would take to lose 50 pounds or more. I have the greatest respect for that person who tries. Of course we know that obese people obviously eat a lot to get as big as they are but more often than not, they become closet eaters. In other words, in front of us it may look as though they don't eat much. They eat less in front of others because they know the jokes and smart remarks about them will come out. They much prefer to eat quietly behind closed doors.

I remember a student nurse in my nurses' training class years ago did just that. She was such a loner and was by far the heaviest of the whole student body. There were five of us in our little click. We studied together, went out on Friday nights together, and ate together. To watch

Joanie eat, you would think she was on a diet because she ate very little in front of us. On study nights, we would often take turns going to each other's rooms for a change, and Joanie would never let us in her room. When we would meet for weekend outings, and she wasn't ready yet, which was usually the case, I'd knock on her door and she still would never let me in. She barely opened the door and said she'd be right out or she'd be a little late and would catch up with us. Sometimes she would, but most of the time she never showed.

One weekend, after we all decided to go out on a pretty autumn Sunday afternoon, I knocked on Joanie's door, as usual, and told her we were ready to go. I didn't get an answer and I was concerned since I hadn't seen or heard from her since the day before. The others wanted to go anyway, so I told them to go ahead and I would go check on Joanie. I got the house mother to open the door and inside there was blood everywhere. Joanie had tried to commit suicide by slashing her wrists. I thought she was dead, but she was just unconscious and ended up in the hospital for several days.

Part of me wasn't surprised with what happened, but when you are young and have yet to experience something like that, it was extremely upsetting to say the least. They found so much junk food that there was enough to have a convenience store, and her closet and drawers were stuffed with every type of sweets and junk food imaginable. Her father came to take her home for a while, but later on she had dropped out, and we never heard from her again. To this day, I often think about her and the personal hell she must have been living. The rest of us were the typical giggling, teasing nineteen-year olds, cute, mostly slender, and as boy-crazy as teenagers are at that age.

Perhaps, had I been into exercise in those days rather than boys, I might have been able to help her get outside of her self-torment. There are so many young people today who live in a tormented state over boys, grades, or just competition with each other about their weight and looks. They turn to food because it is so comforting when society isn't. If we could spend more time trying to understand what really goes on in an overweight person's mind, perhaps we can help turn their lives around where they realize the good in themselves rather than just the good in food.

> "More people in the US die of eating too much rather than too little."— John Galbraith, *The Affluent Society*

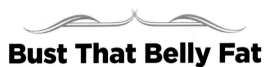

Bust That Belly Fat

You are in a hurry to lose some weight, but dieting has never worked in the past plus the fact that you have very little will power, so you are reluctant to diet again. Here are a few helpful hints to get you started gradually, and these will ensure losing at least five pounds without so much sacrifice.

1. At the very least, cut down your sugar intake and I don't just mean table sugar but cookies, candy, etc. For instance, instead of eating 2 donuts in the morning, eat one if you have to.instead of having a bag of chips with your take out sandwich at subway, skip the chips.in the evening, instead of eating your whole dinner, leave a few tablespoons of the potatoes or rice on your plate instead of in your mouth. For a night time snack, don't eat something sweet like a few pieces of candy or cookies, eat a pear or dish of strawberries. Another alternative, eat a protein bar. These suggestions are just that, suggestions. Any time you eat a little less daily at each meal without changing your regular

diet you can and will lose a few pounds at a slower rate but you will lose. I recommend this to those who refuse to diet but want to be a little thinner. This is a great way to help your mindset get into a less is more mode.

2. Another great trick, simple but efficient, cut out any fats in your regular diet, ie, if you ordinarily cook with olive oil use, "smart choice" spray on instead of "pam". Instead of adding butter as flavor to veggies or meat, you "I can't believe it's not butter," a few squirts; instead of regular salad dressing, use light and stick with the amount listed on the bottle as serving size; if you are having pasta, limit the amount of pasta, add steamed veggies to the pasta, then use "classico "tomato based marinara sauces. By the time you mix this all together you actually have plenty of pasta without getting that stuffed feeling. The trick is eliminating oil or butter for flavor because you can. When you see the difference in the scale after a week of doing this you will realize you really can go without even the so called healthy fats. I recommend this for those of you who are so used to using olive oil and butter a lot. Even the so called "healthy" fats are still fat, remember that a tablespoon of oil has 14 grams of fat. Who stops at a tablespoon? Just constantly keep in mind that fat calories are 3 times harder to burn off than sugar calories (carb calories). I'm not saying to go out and eat lots of sugary foods. You need to cut both but of the 2 fat is far more important to cut out.

3. A really fast weight loss trick but one of the hardest to do is eliminate everything in your diet that has salt or sodium in it. Remember as you read the nutrition labels on the packages, that sodium means salt. When you start to add up all the sodium in everything that we eat, ie, breast of chicken, a slice of cheese, frozen vegetables, etc there is a substantial amount of sodium in it. Sodium always will retain fluid and 1 teaspoon of salt, even sea salt, garlic salt in addition to regular table salt will cause your body to hold 2 extra pounds of weight period. It's imperative to watch your salt content especially for those of you who love salt! When I was growing up in the 60's we loaded everything with salt. I can remember my mother adding salt to just about everything that she cooked. Then at the dinner table, we would pass around the salt shaker. Sadly, to this day I do love salt and salty pretzels and chips. I do eat these sparingly because I know the salt not only affects the taste but health conditions as well, such as high blood pressure which can lead to other problems. If you get in the habit of using natural herbs and at least the powders, such as garlic, or onion powder, you will be much better off. This does take some adjustment especially for people like me who grew up eating a lot of salt. Salt, unfortunately does add a lot of taste to foods but that really can change by adding some of the flavorful herbs out there. Once you get used to adding herbs and salt free spices, you won't want

to go back to salt It's interesting to me, if I have something that does have a lot of salt in it after not having much salt for awhile, you can really taste the difference, more often than not you can't handle the additional salt. Try it for awhile and you'll see the difference.

4. Another bust the belly fat trick is eat lots and lots of watermelon especially when it is in season and so reasonable.It is an outstanding fruit that satisfies the sweet craving, is low in calories, and fills you up and not out! In fact, years ago there was the "beverly hills diet." For 3 days you ate nothing but watermelon. The problem is you got so much gas from the watermelon, it is best not to be around anyone you liked. The good news is you are so full from the water content (and gas I might add!) That it took away the desire to eat anything else let alone anything fattening. You can drop 10 pounds in 3 days with this little tip so if you need to lose a fair amount of weight fast to get into a certain dress or go to a big function this definitely works.

5. Do you like bagels, lox, and cream cheese? This is a great belly buster in limited amounts. To this day I still eat bagel and lox at least once a week for lunch or for my dinner when I don't feel like cooking.the lox provides substantial protein and omega 3 oil definitely use the whipped or light cream cheese over regular to cut the calories and fat content in half.what's great is that this combination is so satisfying, you stay satisfied

for hours.if you add a little lemon that's a bonus since lemon is a diuretic and a fat burner as well. The point is always try to use the substances that enable your body to do the work, ie increase metabolism and burn fat.

By now, you know that some fats are good for you and necessary for our bodies to work well. We do actually need a small amount of fat in our diet every day to stay well tuned, so to speak. But if you are on a fat free diet as many are today, it is best to get as little fat as possible in our foods. that small amount of fat that our bodies do need daily will also take some of our desire for sweets away so it really is a double edge sword. Fat in very small amounts is ok.

Regarding your love of sweets, all sugar does turn to fat, sorry but it's true.you may even have a sugar addiction which does take significant will power to overcome, I know because I'm still trying! A sugar addiction is actually as strong as a drug addiction and is almost as difficult to overcome.the average person consumes 1,000 times the amount of sugar in all its forms than what the body needs. The down side, it definitely contributes to excess belly fat, gives a false pancreatic reading which puts stress on insulin production so the excess is stored as fat.

An emotion that contributes greatly to excess belly fat is stress, the anxiety you feel leads to excessive cortisol production internally which creates more belly fat by slowing down your metabolic rate. Usually this fat is stored right around the abdomenal area and once again is difficult to lose. Until you get your stress level under control it will be difficult to get rid of. This cortisol literally causes the body to store fat rather than burn it off. It's like a savings account in a way, the body needs extra fat stores when your insulin production slows down and it does this with the secretion of cortisol which you don't need or want. Until you learn to relax excessive cortisol will be formed.

6. At least twice a day of completely relaxing or destressing, could mean an inch off your belly in a short period of time. Why wouldn't you want to do it?

7. Taking a calcium tablet every day also helps decrease belly fat. We are so used to hearing about bone health that we overlook another main function of calcium and that is to start the whole fat burning process in the body. Show me a really chubby person and I'll show you someone who doesn't take daily calcium even if that person drinks milk.

8. On occasion have that glass of wine. That 4 ounce. glass of wine is actually better for you than a 12oz soda. Soda actually sends your metabolism into a frenzy just as daily coffee does. It's actually the caffeine which causes havoc with the blood sugar level which in turn makes you want to eat more.

"My grandmother started to walk five miles a day at the age of sixty. She's now ninety-seven and we don't know where the heck she is!"—Ellen Degeneres

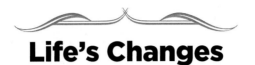

Life's Changes

Whenever you have a major change in your life, there typically is a weight gain or loss. Unfortunately, 75% of the time there is weight gain. How many of you mothers out there noticed when your children were infants or toddlers you found it impossible to keep your weight under control in spite of constantly running after them? In fact, your sleep deprivation due to your having to get up a few times a night to tend to your baby causes your metabolism to plummet. Although you are tired, you have to keep going, and as a result, you start to gain a few extra pounds. As your toddler grows and explores every nook and reachable cabinet in the house, you tend to grab snacks not just for the little one but also for yourself. Then you grabbed a few cookies or pop tarts or anything that was easily within reach and you thought would give you some energy to get you through the rest of the day, and before you knew it, you already gained another couple of pounds. And you still look pretty good in jeans, so you don't worry about it, even though your jeans are beginning to get a little snug.

Before long, the child is four years old and you are also twenty pounds heavier. Statistically, if you don't lose your post-baby weight by the time your baby is a year old, you're bound to be overweight for the rest of your life. You have to realize this all started with too little sleep and too much snacking more than anything else, but the good news is that you can curb the weight gain if you start now, not tomorrow or next week but now.

At times when you feel so exhausted that it is hard to even keep your eyes open, you tend to grab something quick to nibble, as I've done millions of times throughout my life. And since you don't want to get even more overweight than you already are, you force yourself to try to do something about it.

So here's a tip, when you are so tired you can't stand it, do jumping jacks or run in place for a few minutes. Little by little you will find yourself starting to feel more energetic. While your child is napping, put on some fast music. That will perk you up instantly and before you know it, you'll be humming and dancing to the beat. You can get a half hour of exercise without even realizing it. The best thing is now you don't feel so tired and sluggish. Soon, you'll be looking forward to the child's nap time because it will become your "me" time. As the weather gets warmer after the child's nap you'll enjoy putting the child in its stroller and getting some fresh air. You'll both love it. I always feel better when I'm outside in nature.it really gets tiresome indoors with either a heater or an air conditioner going all the time.fresh air does wonders for our bodies and our skin.

Another big change in a person's life is when you leave home for the first time. You are no longer under the rule of your parents whether you are college bound, or working and getting your first apartment. How I remember those days! No one is there to criticize every morsel of food you eat. Typically you feel such freedom because you can eat whatever you want and whenever you want.like most young people on their own for the first time, you tend to eat a lot of pizza, hamburgers and fries, lots of fattening snacks, donuts in the a.m. to get you going and chips and sodas to end your day.remember, since I've been there and done that how well I know.as a result, the pounds start coming on and don't seem to stop. You once had a great body, and even though it is still great, your friends say you are pleasingly plump or round, firm, and fully packed.I know because I was told that early on for years and thought it was ok to look that way. Little did I understand the truth years ago.

My very first time away from home, I was studying to be a registered nurse. We as student nurses could eat all the food we wanted when we wanted at the student cafeteria or medical staff dining room. There was even a subterranean dining room for after hour students and employees of the hospital. There were many nights, while studying, I would go down there and eat nothing but high calorie, nutritionless meals and desserts. To make a long story short, I packed on the pounds.

Often times people gain weight when they are newlyweds because as a young wife you want to please your husband so you try all these great recipes. Of course, the down side to that, in addition to eating these terrific smelling and tasting dishes, you tend to taste them as you go along. And what happens, you and your new husband start to look like little butterballs!

The next big change of course, is midlife, as the woman goes through menopause. Typically, the kids are on their own now so you can relax a lot more and at times, both you and your husband get a little lazy. You might travel more, go out a little more often, and not only does your metabolism slow down as you get older but so do your exercise habits.as we lose more muscle mass, we get more flabby. I've seen too many people who just laugh and say, "I'm getting older so I'm slowing down." I say," stop right there and absolutely don't buy into that!" You can change that and be as young acting and physical as you want to be. In my 60's I'm far more active and fit than I was in my 20's and I have no intention of slowing down. I like looking and feeling good. I'm vain, I admit it. You can keep your lean muscle mass and little to no flab if you keep on moving! It takes only an hour a day and out of a 24 hour day what is one simple hour? I'll tell you what it is, it is high energy, great muscle tone, little to no belly fat, low cholesterol, low blood pressure, flexible joints, ie, no stiffness. Shall I go on? I certainly would rather give up an hour for exercise than to have all of that plus flab. Wouldn't you?

There is no other way around it. "move it to lose it!"

One of the most difficult life change that may hit home with you, is the break up of a relationship be it a husband, soulmate, or partner. I, who am often referred to as the energizer bunny, want to share this story with you. I was happily involved in a long term relationship for years. I thought we were basically happy and everyone said what a great couple we were, always the life of the party, had tons of friends, and life couldn't be better. Then one day, while out on his boat on the island of maui where we lived blissfully, he said, "carol, I need some space. I care about you but really need some space that I never had since my wife died and you came into my life." He went on to say he wanted me to move out as soon as possible. Luckily, I owned a condo in florida so went there since I couldn't stand the thought of staying on maui where he was and all our friends were. Those of you who have gone to the hawaiian islands know what a small community the outer islands are. My initial reaction was that I got physically ill, went down to 104 pounds because I couldn't think about food, even my favorite dishes. This went on for months and I thought I would never feel happy again. I didn't even want to exercise, I just wanted to sleep as often as I could. Then one morning, it hit me. I forced myself out of bed and started walking. I walked for miles because the walking definitely helped ease the pain of loss. The mere fact of being outside in this beautiful area by the sea, I began to feel good again. Also my appetite came back with a vengeance, darn it! The point of the story isn't my appetite but to let you know that often times one can lose too much weight which can be as harmful to you as gaining weight. The joy is knowing that the dark days pass, and the light shines again. You can and will move on. It really is the walking that got me through the down times. Little by little, I felt whole again and started meeting other people. Now, I look back and think it was a great experience and I grew from the experience. As the pain of loss dwindles, the healing takes over as well your sense of well being. Isn't time wonderful? It is the great healer if you allow it to be.

No matter what changes occur in your life, whether they be emotional or not, understand that they do have an impact on your lifestyle. This includes sleeping, eating and physical habits. The good news is that we have the ability to overcome these difficult times. No matter how impossible it seems at the time to get through "changes," with faith and strength, we can move on.the other benefit of getting out of your chair and start moving is that exercise will quicken your emotional healing, once those endorphins start kicking in you will feel great again.

> "Losing weight isn't a walk in the park, but once you lose it, you'll love walking in the park."—Carol Dexter

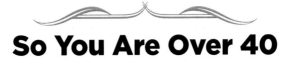

So You Are Over 40

I always have to chuckle when I read horror stories about people over 40 and especially women. It is as though society thinks we are going to dry up and wither away. You can buy into whatever you want to buy into but please do as I do, laugh about it all.

Yes, it's true that your metabolism does slow down after forty. In fact, your metabolic rate drops 5% every ten years. You can eat basically the same foods, try to watch your weight, exercise a little every day buy you are starting to get that flabby belly you never had before. Your upper arms start to wiggle, thighs and buttocks start to look like jello, and you just say, "help!". As you age, a slower metabolic rate means that your body burns far fewer calories than it did when you were in your twenties and thirties. Also, your estrogen level starts to decline, and your body increases the number of fat cells to make up for the decreased production of estrogen. Because fat cells burn fewer calories than muscle cells, this too decreases your metabolic rate, hence, the weight gain. If you are eating exactly the same as before you will gain weight. This happens because the insulin production increases, sending sensors to your appetite center saying you are hungry, which increases body fat that leads to inflammation and increase in the desire for food. When you eat more to feel full, you feel fatigue because by this time you can't sleep well at all. And because you don't sleep well, you are tired and don't have the energy to do much of anything, let alone exercise. Also, your thyroid level drops, which increases hunger and adds to your deep belly fat that's starting to get difficult to lose.

The bottom line is that you have to start moving. When you move, your muscle mass starts to come alive again. The more muscle you have in your body, the better your metabolism works, and the better the metabolism works, the quicker you will lose weight. Muscle burns three times more calories than fat.

There are so many simple ways to fight flabby bellies, arms, and thighs, but you have to really want to lose that flab. A woman is far more attractive to men if they have firm muscles and just a few wrinkles. First of all, cut out as much fat and sugar from your diet as you can. Stop frying food, it never does any good, even once in a while. Drink Oolong green tea, at least three cups a day, and I guarantee you that you will become a fat-burning machine. You can actually burn up to 35% more fat a day just by drinking unsweetened green tea. Also, it's loaded with antioxidants, which will help prevent the free radicals that cause illness. Pepper acts as a metabolic booster, and lemon is a natural diuretic to help you get rid of the toxins that your body has built up hence an excellent choice is lemon pepper should you like both pepper and lemon.

Cinnamon also speeds up metabolism. Drink lots of water, iced water, the colder the better. Eight glasses a day will burn off up to seventy calories! Pineapple is another wonderful fat burner, so much so, that its bromelain extract is used in countless thermogenic products on the market to help your body cut down on inflammation and increase fat burning.

Another trick, at the very least, trim off one hundred calories a day to lose several pounds a year. I know it sounds like a long term, but by just shaving some calories here and there and adding exercise, just imagine how trim you'll become. Instead of butter, use Smart Choice or other low fat butter, use light salad dressings and yogurts instead of the regular ones, add sour cream to baked potatoes instead of butter, or better yet get the steamer bags of broccoli in light cheese sauce instead of butter altogether. You may have some other ideas where to trim a few calories. You may also increase your daily protein intake; there are great protein bars and shakes in the market if you are in a hurry and don't have time to sit down and eat to help increase it. I personally now like frozen yogurt instead of ice cream, and that has 50% fewer calories and fat. Another great trick is to slow down, take your time and savour every bite. You'll find that you'll actually get satisfied with far less than you would normally eat., Also, before you sit down to watch TV, grab two one-pound cans of veggies(or light weights if you have them), sit down and relax, and then with a can in each hand, slowly raise your arms, then bring them back down by bending your elbows to waist level, and raise and lower again fifteen times. Do this in sets of two and increase to three in a few days. Do the same number of squats for your thighs and lunges (one leg forward) for your abs. Do all three of these easy exercises daily and you will be absolutely amazed at the changes in your muscle tone, which in effect will start to decrease your weight. Every movement you make, every extra little thing will all help you in your weight battle, regardless if you are forty, fifty, or seventy years old! Just do it and what a better day to start than now.

Be kind to your body no matter your age, because your body is the best investment you ever have. Always remember, there are only two ways to lose weight: eat fewer calories than your body needs, and eat the same but increase your daily exercise. If you prefer to do the latter, you will lose a pound a week on an average, but at least, you lose.

> "Exercise is the average working person's answer to plastic surgery!"—Author unknown

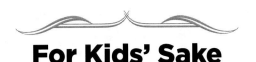

For Kids' Sake

After working forty hours all week, dropping off and picking up the kids from school, then helping them with their homework when you'd much rather watch TV for a change, Saturday has finally arrived. You can actually sleep in until almost eight o'clock while the kids are spread out in front of the television; that will keep them occupied for hours. When you do get up, you fix them a pop tart and a glass of milk, which they barely acknowledge because their eyes are glued to the cartoon channel. You take this time to do some housecleaning and laundry, or maybe not because it is Saturday and you finally get to relax a little. By noon, the cartoons are over, so you make peanut butter and jelly sandwiches for lunch and a few cookies for dessert. The kids quickly gobble down their food and run back to the living room to watch more television. By mid afternoon, you tell them to turn the television off because you are all going on some errands. They of course, moan and groan but still turn the TV off, although reluctantly anyway.

Imagine this scenario instead: the children still get to watch an hour or so of cartoons so that you can quickly straighten up the house. Then you come back into the living room in workout shorts and top, or just something comfy to do a little exercise in. Your little darlings look at you momentarily like you are a stranger in their home, and as you walk over to the TV and turn it off, you say, "Come on, kids, let's go take a walk to the park." Now they look at you as though you are crazy and say, "But we always drive. It's too far to walk." Really, it is only three blocks away, which is one reason why you bought the house in the first play. You visualized the countless hours the children would delight in playing there, but it never worked out that way, thanks to TV and computer games. They never want to get off the couch.

Just imagine, as a mother, what a positive effect your child will have in seeing you do something active. Don't be afraid to get your child started at a very young age, three or four even, whether it be taking a short walk with the dog or going to the park to play on the swings and slide. When you see an overweight parent, 90% of the time the child will be overweight as well. If you tend to be sedentary at home, so will your child be. The child becomes a chubby teenager, is ridiculed at school all the time, which generally causes them to become a loner. He or she is much more comfortable sitting around eating and watching TV.

So for your sake and the sake of the child, stop that cycle. You can do it by taking small steps so it won't be overwhelming to you or your child. You can start by keeping some exercise equipment around, something as simple as a ball, a pair of skates, or a jumping rope. Do whatever you can to encourage movement. You can always set up "an outside play hour" for the family. Get everyone involved, even the dog. Dogs are great play companions. Before you know it, you will all be outside running around, playing tag with each other and laughing. You can also go bike riding with the kids. It is a wonderful way to really see everything. Everything your child does physically well compliment him or her along the way. We all like to be praised; it is a far better reward system for children than always giving them some potato chips or candy when they've done something well. And before long, you'll just find yourself hearing your kids say, "Mommy, watch me." They would also love hearing you say, "That's wonderful, great job." Your approval is paramount. But I'm not telling you anything new; you're the mother after all.

Kids are more likely to stick with something physical they enjoy doing. Their attention span is so limited when they are young that whenever you are teaching them something to learn, you have to keep it fun and verbally rewarding. Years ago, while living in Maui, I, along with several other adults, used to help teach tennis to children. Lahaina, Maui had such a wonderful after-school tennis program. For well under a hundred dollars a year, parents could enter their children into the junior tennis program. As soon as school let out, usually around two thirty, the children would walk across the street to the tennis courts. They would stay there until five o'clock or so.

Essentially, it was a very inexpensive babysitting program for the parents. The kids loved it because they were interacting with other children who liked tennis, and as most children do when they had a few breaks, they would tease and laugh with each other as they drank water or sodas. What I admired were the countless hours, weeks, months, and often years the volunteer adults gave to these children, helping them to learn tennis. Oftentimes it wasn't easy. We would create drills but in such a way that the child wouldn't become bored and say, "I don't want to play anymore, I'm tired." This did happen on a daily basis, especially among the girls around ages eight to ten. I used to try to make it fun and challenging, me against them, and how they would love to think they beat the teacher! The desire to win starts at a very young age. Sometimes I would offer a prize if they could get the ball over the net up to five times in a row, and it was always amazing how, as soon as you said a prize, their interest level would skyrocket.

Be creative with your children. You want to always encourage movement in the form of exercise every day, even for just twenty minutes at a time so that in time they will become conditioned to do it. I love it when I see children say, "Come on, Mom, let's go for a bike ride." Here in Florida, you hear "Can we go to the beach?" all the time. If you don't have children or your children are grown and no longer at home, take some time and go to the beach. It really is fun just watching children at the beach. As soon as they hit the sand from the parking lot, their little legs go into a running mode. They try to head to the water immediately but their parents always say, "Hold on. I have to put sunscreen on you." But something magical comes over them as they reach the surf. You hear shouts of joy and laughter, and it doesn't stop until you make them have a sandwich, which they eat as fast as they can before they once again rush to the shoreline. What a wonderful way to get in exercise, and yet they don't realize it. They just think of it as playing.

It really is so easy to teach children, they will follow because they are so eager to please. As they are growing up, they love to be active. If they aren't, you have to encourage them to be one in a loving way. Because I'm so actively involved in tennis, I do hate to see parents who try to force an activity onto a child. Or yell at the child for not doing something right. As a parent, it is your task to make their exercise time enjoyable because if you don't, chances are the child will rebel against the activity throughout his teen and adult years. Think of yourself as you were growing up. If you didn't have any encouragement to play sports or be active, then you'll have a hard time getting into physical activities all your life. I grew up in a relatively inactive family; however, I think I was born wired for movement. I could never be still, which is a good thing for me. Even up to this day, I wouldn't know what it is like to feel tired. By being active all my life, my metabolic rate hasn't plummeted as I got older.

While living in Hawaii years back, I would always visit my family in Detroit usually at Christmas because it meant a lot to my mother. It was usually too cold to be outside for a long period of time, so I would go into the basement and put on fast music and dance to the music for a couple of hours. When I'd hear my nieces and nephews come to the house, I knew in a few minutes they would come running down the steps to join me in the basement. They thought it was great fun jumping around and dancing to the music. Little did they know that I was trying to teach them positive movement habits. For many days, after a heavy snowstorm, I'd tell the children I was going for a walk in the snow and they eagerly cried, "Can we come?" I looked like the pied piper with four little ones often trailing along with me. It didn't matter that it was cold and snowing, we all loved it.

I was the only one in my family who really liked exercise in any form. Perhaps that's why I tried to encourage it with other children whose parents didn't like to wherever and whenever I could. If only adults would have even some of the enthusiasm that children have, Life for them would certainly be a lot more fun and exciting.

> "If you are going to try cross-country skiing, start with a very small country."—Author unknown

Keep It Simple and Safe

One experience that's definitely wonderful to witness is a baby's growth. In the first few months, she sleeps most of the time, and a little after that she tries to sit up but tends to roll onto her side without the help of the mother. Oftentimes if the infant is on the couch, the mother sets throw pillows on either side of her so that she can sit upright at least momentarily while she takes a picture. A month or so later, the baby attempts to crawl around only to keep rolling over again. When she feels a little stronger, she then attempts to stand up and grins from ear to ear when she realizes she can do it. She may wobble a bit then fall down but she'd keep trying to stand again until she gets it right.

A few years later, the child is about five years of age and wants to learn to ride a bike. You get her a darling pink bike (every little girl seems to want a pink bike with tassels on the handle bar). You make sure the training wheels are in place before she sits and you gently show her how to hold on as she pedals. As soon as you let go, she is thrilled, knowing she can ride all by herself.

Technically, this is no different from an overweight person starting out on an exercise routine. If you think of it as an overwhelming project then that's what it will become, and you'll keep putting it off until next week or after the holidays. You don't have to say, "I'm going to join a gym next week and then I'll start going regularly," because that seldom ever gets done. Next week turns into the following week, and before you know it, three months have passed you by and you still haven't gone. Worse yet is the person who says, "I just joined a gym, so I'm going to go three to five days a week." Generally, out of 10 women I counseled, 9 of them tell me this very same thing, and when I see them a week later, I typically hear, "I just didn't have time to go this week, but I will next week." That same person gets angry because as soon as she stepped on the scale, she was up another three pounds. She becomes angry with herself and angry with the clinic because she didn't lose. Oftentimes when that happens, she is so angry or embarrassed that she stops coming to the clinic for a month or so. When she finally comes back, she's already gained ten or fifteen pounds.

It is basically the same thing with preferring to walk instead of going to a gym. So often I hear people say, "I'm going to walk three miles every day," but the same thing happens. When I counsel the client the next week and ask, "How is your walking doing?" I usually know the answer even before she opens her mouth. Dont' start by walking miles. Walk a block or two. Try to get in twenty minutes a day—ten minutes one way and another ten back. When your body isn't used to exercise, it definitely rebels, so you might get a few aches and pains until your muscles adapt to this new regimen. Keep in mind that those muscles haven't been seriously used for years most likely. God designed us with moveable body parts for a reason, and that's to keep moving! So move, but take things one step at a time. In a week or so, you'll be feeling good again. Start with baby steps; you really do have to crawl before you can walk. Keep that in mind and little by little, you'll start feeling better.

The real trick is to build distance slowly so that your body will adjust. I advise starting out every other day until you are strong enough for a daily routine. Before you know it, you'll start looking forward to that "me" time. It's a chance for you to think or enjoy the sights without phone or family interruptions. Most of us have so much going on in our lives that we use that precious time as meditation time, a time to thank God for life and the ability to enjoy all that is around us.

I'm always so energized that I think of it as my "calming time." I meditate and organize my day during that time, and that alone will refresh me and put me in a better place to start the day. And so will you. When you are able to take the time to walk in the morning, or do whatever form of exercise you prefer, it really helps you to stay on an even keel throughout the day, no matter what crisis comes up. I do prefer the morning for my work out for that reason. However, sometimes, with complications in our schedules, we have to work out at night, which usually leads to us saying, "I think I'll skip today and work out tomorrow instead." Bottom line is, get it in no matter how brief the time span is. It is well worth the sweat.

> "Aerobics is a series of strenuous exercises, which help to convert fats, sugars, and starches into aches, pains, and cramps."—Author unknown

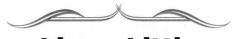

Live a Little

M ost diet and nutrition experts the world over stress the importance of eating the right nutrients and food items for your body; that is, making sure you eat the five basic food groups daily. As you probably know, these include dairy, meat or fish and poultry, whole grains, which of course, are complex carbohydrates, healthy fats such as olive oil, avocados, nuts, and legumes such as beans.

When it comes to dieting or eating to lose weight, instead of insisting you munch on celery and carrot sticks when you are hungry, I say, "live a little" and eat a treat. Please don't get me wrong, I'm not saying you go ahead and eat whatever you want all the time, because that would defeat your purpose, which is to lose weight and get into shape. By making some basic changes in your eating habits and setting aside at least a half hour a day to get up and start moving, you will also become slimmer and be able to enjoy those treats!

Man is created beautifully with lots of moveable parts, so keep them moving. Think about it, our cars need gas, oil, and proper maintenance to keep working, and it's the same with our bodies. Being able to move is one of life's greatest pleasures. I surely don't want my body to break down and come to a stop just because I'm too lazy to take care of it with routine maintenance.

Picture a person you may have seen recently in a wheelchair, or a person too crippled to even walk by themselves across a busy street. Have you ever been sick or bedridden after surgery, for instance, and thought to yourself, "If only I could get up and walk to the bathroom." Believe me, I've been there, post-op, and it is not pleasant.

I was in church one Sunday not long ago, and a woman sitting in front of me cried out because she couldn't even make it to the altar for communion. There are thousands and thousands of people who have illnesses or conditions and would give anything in the world to be able to move again, if just for a moment. Just how lucky we healthy people are! For these people, to "live a little" would mean something different entirely.

> "Don't dig your grave with your own knife and fork."—english proverb

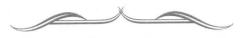

If You Don't Use It, You Won't Lose It

Stop thinking of exercise as a major drudgery. A great way to make it a major part of everyday life is doing small things at first that require body movement. Remember a baby's first steps before he learned to walk? This is no different. First, the baby rolls over, then a few weeks later he learns to sit up without rolling onto his side; then he learns to crawl, on to standing up holding onto something firm, and finally, he starts to walk.

It is no different for a person who has never really exercised in his life. First, you walk about ten minutes in one direction, then ten minutes back. Every week you add another ten minutes and some speed. Eventually, you'll be looking forward to that hour break from being a mom, wife, or girlfriend, and you just enjoy nature around you. If you are in the city, that's a great time to window-shop or check out the neighborhood. When it is too hot outside, do a shopping center stroll. You can do a mile or two in no time.

Another idea, don't drive around for ten minutes waiting for a parking spot right in front of the store to become available. Save gas and money by parking at the end of the row. Your body will thank you for all those little ways to exercise, I guarantee it. And if you have a dog that needs walking, do it. Dogs absolutely love to go outside. As soon as I would pick up my dog's leash, she would be so excited she'd turn around in circles and wiggle her behind so much that I would often have a hard time getting her leash on her. It just takes a few extra blocks a day to help your pet and you. And don't rush back as soon as your pet has gone to the bathroom, let him sniff around a little. That's the nature of the animal, so don't deprive the dog of what it enjoys doing during those few minutes it is outside with you.

One of the most upsetting things for me to see is a family pet that is grossly overweight. Usually where there is a chubby dog, there is a chubby owner behind who merely lets his dog out to do its business then brings it back in as soon as it's done. The other frustrating thing is to see a house with a doggie door. The owner doesn't have to move and walk the dog around, although he probably might need the exercise but is just too lazy to have the time to walk the dog. I know there are times when we are in such a hurry because we didn't allow enough time for the dog or yourself so you do scramble, trying to fit in a quick walk for your pet. I know, I've definitely been there.

According to many top choreographers and professional dancers, part of their daily routine is to squeeze their butt muscles for five seconds at a time, fifteen repetitions, two sets, and they would be doing this four times a day. This simple mini exercise alone will help tone your butt, and there likely aren't any excuses not to be able to do this certain exercise, since you can just do this while sitting. In fact, I'm doing this while typing this book! Try this religiously and you'll be amazed how great your butt will look anyway!

If you're at a lecture, in a movie, or in an airplane and have to sit for long periods of time, you can do the flexed leg raises by either bending your leg at the knee or using your whole leg if you have the room. Even establishments find ways to help customers to move. In extreme weather conditions, many of the shopping malls have extended hours before they open so that the shoppers can do their walking inside.It is an excellent opportunity for customers not only to get some exercise but to see what the stores are promoting as well.

Don't worry about what others might think of you as you embark on different ways to exercise.Most people actually look up to you for doing it.

The moral of this chapter is to always take the extra steps and do whatever it takes to get in some additional time moving your body. Stop with all the shortcuts because every time you move, every additional step you take will pay off tremendously.

> "To lengthen your life, shorten your meals."—100 year old proverb

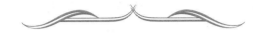

Move Like a Kid Again

While doing an art show in a very posh Maui oceanfront hotel (it wasn't really a show per se, just lots of easels in the lobby displaying the works I had for sale), I couldn't help but notice the small children running around. They never stopped running, and just off the lobby was an expansive Polynesian lawn with lots of palm trees and, of course, the ocean, which made it so inviting for these children to play. There were several waterfalls cascading into natural fish ponds, which complemented the setting.

Children don't understand the difference between walking and running. They are so full of excitement that they can never be expected to stay still even for just a short time. In fact, just in front of where I was stationed, a large family of grandparents, parents, and their children had gathered to pose for a Christmas portrait, and one small child kept leaving the pack, content to be by herself in exploring the koi ponds; she just couldn't stand still long enough for a photo shoot. You could just feel the excitement and energy within this little person. It was such a wonderful sight to behold. The other children were just about as excited, except for one little chubby girl. This child, on the other hand, was quiet, withdrawn, not taking part in the family's festivities but was contentedly munching away on a handful of cookies while holding a bag of chips in her other hand. Interestingly, her mother and father were also chubby. In fact, they were the only other chubby couple out of the four couples. And unless their eating habits and lifestyle start to change soon, that chubby little girl will most likely end up just like them. Go back to being a child again, and I don't mean literally, but feel the joy of movement, running through a waterfall, splashing in the surf, or simply walking along the beach.

For years, everyone blamed overweight conditions on glandular problems. If I had a dollar for every time I heard someone say, "Oh, she has a gland problem, and that's why she's heavy," Then I would have been rich by now. Basically, the only glandular problems to my knowledge that would affect weight loss or gain would have to do with the thyroid. Today, you are simply hypo or hyperthyroid—either you are sluggish and tired all the time, or you are wired and don't like to stop moving. Either way, there are medications that you can take for those conditions, regardless whether you are too thin or too heavy. Most people, however do have normal thyroid function.

Let's face it, 90% of the time, when excessive weight is an issue, laziness and excuses are the issue. if you tend to be that person who gets up in the morning, grabs a bite to eat, gets in the car, drives to work, does the mostly sedentary eight-hour thing, goes home, fixes dinner, watches TV for a few hours, goes to bed, and then repeats that routine day in and day out, of course, you are going to gain weight. Your body is made to move, never forget that. The heavier you get, the harder it is to move. You become more tired, and extra pounds will definitely put an extra strain on your heart, let alone your body and your energy level.

As the cycle continues, you get heavier and heavier to the point where everything becomes all about exerting more and more effort. You probably ache just trying to get out of bed in the morning, or are tired all day and are counting the hours until you're through work so that you can go relax. Your body is a beautiful moving machine, and treating it as such does take an incredible commitment. But once you do, you can act like that glorious child again, a child who enjoys every single movement all the time.

> "The older you get, the harder it is to lose weight because by then, your body and your fat have become good friends."—Anonymous

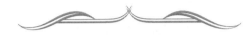

If We Could Bottle Up
That Adrenalin High

How many times in your life have you been so excited when that certain person called and asked you out on a date? Remember that sudden rush you felt, that feeling of overwhelming joy and you could hardly contain yourself? You couldn't wait to call your best friend and tell her the news, and nothing at that moment could bring you down, even food.

Go further back when you were still applying to a college or a job that you wanted so badly. When the acceptance notice or the long-awaited phone call came in, you were so happy you wanted to burst. Again, did you want to run to the refrigerator to go look for something to eat in the heat of the moment? Not a chance. Instead, you felt like shouting on a rooftop, "I got the job!" or "I got accepted!" What a glorious feeling, indeed.

Just take a moment to go down memory lane and think about those wonderful occasions in your life when you felt that way. What was the first thing you wanted to do at that precious moment in your life? I bet that having waited for months to hear the words you've dreamt of hearing, you could care less about eating. As the adrenaline was surging through your body, you couldn't stand still; you just had to move! Even as you called your best friend to share the good news, you were probably pacing back and forth.

Whenever I received really exciting news, I made it a point to go out for a brisk walk or jogging. I felt as though I would literally explode with excitement, and the last thing I wanted to do was sit around.

Just imagine, if someone could come up with "bottled natural adrenaline," every person alive would buy it. And of course, the chemist who discovered it would become the wealthiest person in the world. Just think, bottled adrenalin would have no side effects, only positive effects, you would lose weight because you wouldn't feel like eating, exercise like crazy, and you would always be smiling, how great would that be? Oh to have that magic elixir that we all dream about for even a day!

While I was still working in a fairly high-end art sales company in Maui a few years back, our director would often tell us to visualize something tangible that we've always wanted. I'd always wanted a Jaguar (the car, not the cat), and we were to imagine we had the money to buy that item. We were to put a picture of that desired item somewhere we would see it several times a day. Of course, I put the picture on my refrigerator at home then put another picture on my personal drawer at work. The key was to be able to look at the item as many times as possible throughout the day, every day, until we made it a realization. I never did get the Jaguar, but I did increase my sales dramatically, and as a retail business, that was the goal of the experiment. I was only one of eight sales consultants who were all quite competitive. End result, gallery sales nearly tripled over a four-month period.

It's amazing how the mind works. If there is something that you really desire, you can achieve it. At the very least, it takes you out of a negative frame of mind and into a positive one. No matter where this is applied, it becomes a winning situation. I'm not suggesting that you run around the house putting up photos of a slim lady, or you at a thinner time in your life, although it might actually help you to get there again. That little exercise alone just might get you to feel excited enough to want to make it work. When you become excited, your adrenaline kicks into gear, and you're on the road again.

You can have that wonderful, joyous feeling. One of the simplest ways to achieve it is when you are trying to lose ten pounds. You've really worked on changing your eating habits, you are eating more veggies and far less fat and sugar, you're getting into a light exercise routine like walking through the nearby park or taking one more complete stroll around the shopping center because it's cold outside. Then there comes a day when you have to weigh in, but with eyes shut tightly you reluctantly step on the scale, because you are afraid to look after those days of hard work. Suddenly, you do look and then you hear yourself screaming. Your face lights up, and you shout, "I did it, I lost eleven pounds!" Then you run to the closet to try on that beautiful dress you bought months ago because you just had to have it, even though it didn't fit. And when you do, you find that it now fits perfectly, and you don't think you could possibly be any happier at that moment. You are so thrilled you prance around in front of the mirror and look at yourself at every angle. Your adrenalin is at full force and you felt such a surge of joy you wanted to sing a loud!

Everyone can have it time and time again. Setting small attainable goals helps to make it possible, and as you attain those goals, reach a little higher, but take time to celebrate and cherish that moment. Even the smallest of goals will give you that adrenaline rush, that feeling that you can accomplish anything. Those are some of the wonderful blessings of life. Put on great music and dance around the living room. It may look strange and ridiculous, but when you feel that excited and start moving around, you don't even think of it as exercise anymore. Every movement you make will help you to achieve that weight loss you've been working so hard on.

We all have rhythm; some of us just show it better than others. For example, working at a weight loss clinic a few years ago, we held a meeting once a month to have the clients share some of their weight loss success stories. One night, the staff decided to surprise the twenty people who were there by bringing in a Zumba dance instructor. If you have never heard of Zumba, it's a popular and fast exercise routine done to Latin American music. There were a few very overweight, stiff women who said they couldn't take part because they just couldn't move. The beautiful thing that happened was that as the instructor was showing everyone some of the moves to the music, the women were laughing as they were trying to get the hang of it, and slowly, these 3 women who said they couldn't do it started to get up one by one and began moving to the beat. In the end, they all had such a great time, smiling and enjoying the rhythm.

So you see, even those people who feel they can't actually can. How you get yourself into the exercise is but a state of mind. So give a healthy lifestyle a chance, and before you know it, you might already even be enjoying the ride.

> "When a friend tells you look absolutely fantastic, smile and say thanks! It is not the time to be humble. You worked hard and deserve every compliment you get. Be proud of how you look."—Carol Dexter

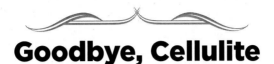

Goodbye, Cellulite

Almost 90% of women particularly suffer from cellulite. Cellulite is the unsightly puckered skin that people have typically around the thigh areas. This flabby look is due to the weakening of the top layer of skin on our thighs particularly the back side, which causes the inner layer to bulge randomly. This is often referred to as the "cottage cheese" look or "orange peel." Women tend to get it more so then men do because in women the connective tissue beneath the skin has more stretch to it. Cellulite always accumulates in our fatty reserve areas, not just in the thighs but also on the back side of upper arms, buttocks, belly, and breasts. Women who are overweight aren't the only people with this problem. Thin people can also have cellulite, particularly if they don't exercise or drink enough water-flavored teas such as raspberry, mango, or even the green teas, which help flush out the cellulite. Drinking at least two quarts of water a day is beneficial in so many ways, and this is one of them.

Foods that contribute the most to forming cellulite are sugar, dairy, meat, and refined white flour products. Dairy products such as yogurt, cheese, butter, sour cream, ice cream, and whipped cream are actually the worst offenders. In addition, red meats rank really high on the list of offenders.

When a person has a sedentary job, chances are that person does not get adequate exercise. It causes a slower digestive process, which can lead to constipation and a much slower metabolism. Because she may have poor elimination, not only do fatty deposits build up but so do toxins. When this happens, the kidneys and liver don't burn off waste efficiently. Most of these problems can be eliminated by, in part, moving around whenever possible. Just about everything we consume turns to fat, and it's why the human body has to move in order to burn it. It literally affects every aspect of our being. Another downside of the lack of body movement is depression, which now affects your emotional state. When you start moving, your body starts to detoxify, thus cutting down the problems that can and will develop if you don't act on it as soon as possible.

There are literally hundreds of products and treatments available to aid in the reduction of cellulite such as creams, lotions, body wraps, pills, to name a few. The creams and lotions act as thermogenic elements, which burn fat to help lessen the appearance of the cellulite. There are no substantiated studies that prove these products actually work, but every body is different in terms of how it reacts to anything we use. If the product seems to work for you, then that is what should count.

There are treatments such as massage, liposuction, laser, and contouring that are an attempt to smooth out the skin. Many of the treatments available are quite costly with no guaranteed results, but there are some that are extremely effective. Always research the product or treatment you want to try and make sure it is the one for you. I would read testimonies, the percentage of good results, and the potential side effects of the product.

Another great trick to rid your body of cellulite is by eating at least 6 to 8 ounces of pineapple every day. Pineapple helps the skin get that smooth, firm look, prevents inflammation after surgery, and is naturally an outstanding fat burner in general. Due to the sugar content and actual makeup of pineapple, it also aids in cutting down your desire for sweet treats. It's interesting that this Polynesian fruit works in that way more so than many other sugar-laden fruits. Try freezing some pineapple chunks then add the frozen form to a protein shake with ice, and you will have one of the tastiest, satisfying drinks in the world!

Aside from pineapple, other most water-based fruits such as watermelon, honeydew, crenshaw, and berries also aid in getting rid of cellulite. You can also blend a package of sugar-free Jell-O, a half cup of frozen fruit, one-and-a-half cups of water, and a half cup of ice, and you'll get a smoothie that is not only refreshing and satisfying but is also definitely working.

Frankly, there is no magic cure that will instantly reduce cellulite. Diet and exercise alone will do wonders for most people. As I stated before, drink lots of water and eat lots of water-based fruits, whole grain foods, and fish.

A more calorie-laden cellulite buster is a slice of whole grain toast with peanut butter, a hard-boiled egg, and a calcium-fortified juice for breakfast. This combination is excellent in breaking down the pockets of dimpled skin.

Try to stay away from fat dense foods, which include fried foods and excessively sugary products. These will only aggravate cellulite, so you would want to stay away from candy, cookies, and other refined flower and sugar items.

But again, exercise is the best cure of all. Think of the money you'll save if you just get into a simple regimen of walking, biking, swimming, among others, instead of spending hundreds of dollars for a so-called "quick fix." A quick fix just doesn't exist; you have to work for it.

> "On jogging or walking, never think how far you have to go, but how far you've come."—Carol Dexter

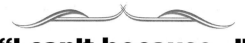

"I can't because..."

I can't because.... I would wager a bet that sometime in your life you have used these excuses, and of course, at that moment you consciously or subconsciously felt it was a legitimate reason not to do any work out or exercise. Here they are:

"I'm anemic, so I get too tired to exercise."

There are only few people in the world who are truly anemic, and those who are can usually control and improve anemia through medication.

"I have a glandular problem, which is why I'm fat and can't move."

Haven't we already analyzed that problem?

"I have an underactive thyroid and don't have enough energy to exercise."

It never ceases to amaze me how many people today buy into this and continue to use this as an excuse when they can simply take meds to change this immediately. Unfortunately, everyone who is substantially overweight blames everything and everyone else for their obesity instead of really being true to themselves and taking the blame. If they would at least admit it is their own fault, that would be a major step in their wanting to change and do something about it. Like I said, the minute you start moving the more energy you will have. Life only gets better!

Yes, it is a major effort but so is changing your sheets, or doing laundry, or even taking out the garbage. You know how difficult it is to start an older car that's been sitting in your grandparents garage for months, well, why should your body be any different? It too gets stiff and creaky from lack of use. No, getting up and going to the refrigerator during commercial breaks definitely don't count as exercise. But then of course, when you don't use all those wonderful parts, you'll be stiff and would rather just sit.

"I can't because I have a bad back and my knees hurt."

So do I. I have a bad back, and the six orthopedic surgeons that I've gone to say that if I don't continue to exercise, it will get worse, so I keep on moving. I probably would have been in a wheelchair by now had I not been exercising all these years because of my degenerative lumbar problem. If I can do it despite the discomfort, so can you. Your mind starts to play wonderful tricks while exercising that you become so focused on what you are doing and temporarily forget about the pain.

When you are overweight, however, your sore knees become worse, and you tend to want to favor the knees and sit because that takes the pressure off the knees. I say if it becomes that uncomfortable to stand or walk, get into a pool—it doesn't even have to be really deep—hold onto the sides and kick your legs, and I promise you they will feel better. Remember, it always takes a little pain to have even a slight gain, but what's important is it does work.

"I can't because I have arthritis."

Do you honestly think your arthritis is going to calm done on its own? It won't, but it just takes for you to get up and move around to control it. For the last thirty-five years, I've been playing a lot of tennis and I hope to keep playing for the next thirty-five years or more. The finger that wraps around my tennis racquet is already getting slightly enlarged from painful arthritis. It hurts a lot for about the first thirty minutes that I'm playing, but I know the pain will lessen dramatically when I work through it, so I just deal with the pain. If we all stop doing the physical things we love to do because of a little pain, no one would play sports anymore. Years ago, when I sold orthopedic prosthetics(knee, shoulder, and hip replacements), many of the physicians told me that the professional athletes who play for a living live in constant and often very severe pain but keep going because that is what they do for a living. Can you imagine what serious pain most athletes are in constantly? I guess I can deal with a little nagging pain, and I'm sure you can too. I know it isn't easy at first, but our bodies are capable of a lot of punishment and mend! Think about it, whenever you see older people who keep moving in those ads on TV or over the internet, they all seem healthy and happy. I especially love the new AD series that show the kid home from college and saying how boring his parents are as he sits home alone immersed on browsing the internet. All the while, his parents are biking, or canoeing, or laughing and having a wonderful time.

Life does not have to stop at forty. To me, it really begins by then. As we age, we are far more content with ourselves and don't get so caught up in so much stress and anxiety. Don't wait another week or month or year before you start to turn your life around. Life quickly passes by, so jump on the physical bandwagon and start enjoying the body God gave you!

"I can't because I'm so busy from the moment I get up, and I just don't have any extra time in the day."

I say, get up a half hour earlier than usual to start with, put on your sneakers, and take a quick walk before everyone else gets up. There's not a time in the day more wonderful than the early morning. I still marvel at a sunrise, with the sun coming up over the ocean while I'm on my way to work. The innocence of dawn is beautiful. If you are working, use a few minutes of your lunch break for a quick ten-minute walk. It does wonders when you get back into the office. I usually tell people to just take a five-minute break and walk around the building. Do that every hour and you've fitted in almost an hour of walking. While others take their five-minute smoke break, take your walk break, and don't sit. If you still didn't make the time through your day but are able to sit down to watch TV for an hour or two, don't get on the computer because it sucks you right in for hours. Instead, walk up and down the stairs, or do some basic abdominal crunches or sit-ups while you're waiting until the commercial is over.

Years ago when I was still working in downtown Honolulu, I'd meet a friend, and we'd put on our running shoes and briskly walk through the park, which was just nearby, then grab a salad or sandwich on the go. Afterward, we would go back to the office and eat for ten minutes instead of thirty. It was a great time in my life. It was our time to share stories, and we'd get so involved we'd walk a lot longer than we intended. What a time indeed to be able to communicate with friends or meet new ones.

"We do not stop exercising because we grow old, we grow old because we stop exercising"—Author unknown

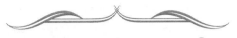

Confessions of a Junk Food Addict

L ike millions of women, I tried virtually every food fad and diet for losing weight while still trying to look great. If it was advertised and seemed to be the popular product at the time, I tried it, including every fat burner, or natural appetite suppressant in the market place in the last 35 plus years.

Years ago when I was still holding sales positions, I had to use my car as my office, driving to a dozen accounts daily. My passion at that time was Dunkin' Donuts, especially the huge fried glazed cinnamon ones. They are so good that I really looked forward each day to my donut treat to kick-start my day. At first, I'd buy just one or two, but soon I started buying a half dozen at a time, thinking they would represent my meals for the day, and all six would be devoured long before I'd call on my last account. I would then take some vitamins once I got home at the end of the day, thinking how bad it could be. I felt so guilty that I'd skip dinner and go for a long run.

Have you ever tried running after eating fried fatty food throughout the day? If not, please don't ever try it. I did, and I got indigestion and then diarrhea. Sometimes I would lose weight and sometimes I wouldn't. The upside though, is that it cured me of my obsession over Dunkin' Donuts. To this day, I haven't been eating them. The point is, you can lose weight on virtually anything as long as you eat less than what your body needs, but that's certainly not a smart thing to do for your body. Then again, when you are young, you try anything that you find might work. And I think that because oftentimes we don't see what really goes on internally, we don't think about the harm these things may do to our bodies.

The opposite of feasting is, of course, fasting. Today, many women, like the models and actresses, are caught up in getting really thin. Unfortunately, this ordeal causes a condition called anorexia, which is a form of self-starvation all for the sake of getting skinny. Anorexia is just as harmful as eating too much, but then again you can't see the damage it does to you internally, so you don't think it is harmful. At that point, you only think about getting thin and staying that way, but anorexia causes a major electrolyte imbalance, severe muscle cramps, vomiting, and irreversible kidney and liver damage, let alone serious heart damage. The overweight person, on the other hand, develops diabetes, high blood pressure, high cholesterol, and too much pressure on the heart to name a few.

First confession: During the holidays, it was a tradition in my family to bake tons of Christmas cookies. When I would go home for Christmas, I looked forward to this tradition, alongside my mother, laughing and talking as we baked. Often, I would starve myself for a week or two before the holiday so that I could eat and bake this wonderful cookie dough, which unfortunately to this day I still enjoy. During the starving phase, I would go to bed so hungry that I would lie there and fantasize about mountains of cookie dough that I would soon be able to consume. Then each morning, I would think, one less day to go until the big cookie bake event!

I would proceed to drop a few heaping spoonfuls of this glorious dough on the baking sheet, then a heaping spoonful in my mouth, and so on and so forth. By about an hour into it, I would be so sick of cookie dough I'd swear I wouldn't eat so much of it ever again. But of course, the next day, I would still do it all over again. The downside, I developed "sugar" headaches, which were as bad as migraines. They would last for hours and hours and no amount of aspirin would get rid of them. The sugar just had to leave the body before these headaches would subside. Now, years later, I realized I was poisoning my body primarily with chocolate and sugar, and that can be very harmful. Now, when I have the urge for cookies, I would buy just one or two that are already baked, so I wouldn't get into trouble. It may not be as fun as those warm memories I had, but I don't miss the headaches, bloated feeling, and the five extra pounds I would gain.

Another confession: Growing up, I used to live across the street from a neighborhood grocery store that had an ice cream counter and sold hand-scooped ice cream for thirty cents a double scoop. Today, a double scoop is around four dollars. But there I was, a preteen, fantasizing about being older on my own and being able to eat all the ice cream I wanted. Today, obviously I am much, much older and still love ice cream, and I don't mean plain boring vanilla. The richer the better, but for weight's and health's sake, I tend to eat light ice cream or frozen yogurt. I still get Cookies and Cream but with much less of the "bad stuff," fats, and calories. I've learned to put it in a cup at home or out rather than a cone or bowl. That way I'll eat a lot less. Not that I don't want more, I do, but I know there are limits to observe in order to keep my weight down.

As you can see, I'm no different than anyone else because I still love to eat, especially dessert! But over time you learn to eat it sparingly. Honestly, when you eat something you love but know that it's fattening and not that good for you, you seem to savor the taste, but in time, you will no longer be desiring it as much as you used to.

Someone once said to me knowing I love cheesecake isn't fattening providing you get enough physical exercise!! The upside is this is true, the downside, it takes running or walking briskly approximately 5 miles to burn off that one slice of cheesecake!

> "If your dog is fat you are not getting enough exercise."—Author unknown, 100 year old proverb

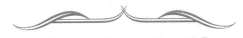

Eat, but Don't Cheat

Here are a few tips that don't make you look as if you are dieting and also work particularly well when you are out.

At a cocktail party or any other kind of party where there is a scrumptious food buffet, don't stand next to a big eater. Research shows we tend to mimic eating habits of those around us. Better to stand next to a slender woman, who is obviously appearance and fashion conscientious. Most likely, she'll nibble on fresh veggies and fruit without the dip. If lots of fresh fruit and veggies and dip are on the table, which is usually the case, eat lots of fruits. Fruits tend to be water-based and very filling, plus the sugar in the fruit tends to prevent you from eating much of the desserts further down the buffet.

Another great party snack to dip into is the cold shrimp platter with cocktail sauce. It's not only really tasty but also full of protein and has no fat. Last year, I was at an event that had huge platters of cold shrimp and crab chilled to perfection. I was in my glory because I love both shrimp and crab, but it is so expensive that I don't often buy it in the grocery stores. But hold off the temptation to dip into butter and creamy sauces. Stay with the tomato-based cocktail sauce, and your figure will love you for it.

If you are in a restaurant, try to eat only grilled chicken, fish, and lean beef. Just watch what you eat with it. Forget the Bernaise sauce or creamy dill sauce for the fish, barbeque sauce for the chicken, and most sauces or marinade for the beef. Grilling itself creates such a wonderful flavor, as do most herbs, lemon, and pepper. Enjoy the baked potato or rice with a small amount of sour cream and chives, but just don't add butter; sour cream is actually much better for you. Plump fresh vegetables al dente or grilled with a splash of lemon and garlic or parmesan make a wonderful side dish and are very filling. If you are having a salad, make it toss greens with a splash of balsamic vinaigrette or other dressing on the side, and dip your greens in it instead of smothering your salad in the dressing. I used to always have a little salad buried in the dressing, and have I changed! Once you get used to less dressing, when you do go out and the restaurant goes overboard on the dressing the salad is no longer flavorful. Try it and you'll become a believer too.

When you are at a lunch meeting or just an outing with your friends, opt for a tuna salad or chicken salad with no dressing on the side, and tell the waiter you can't have too much mayonnaise. Today, people are so aware of what they are eating that restaurants are used to the exceptions and are willing to go the extra mile to please their customers.

Today, the traditional sandwich has been overtaken by the ubiquitous "wrap." You can do anything with a wrap but, the downside is that oftentimes the wrap is made with so much fat that a whole grain bread or roll will be better and much more filling for you for a longer period of time. Places like the subway offer a wonderful variety of fairly low calorie, high protein sandwiches, which are filling.

When cooking at home and preparing dinner that's grilled or baked with lots of herbs and powders such as onion, garlic or even lemon pepper, everyone will enjoy it without the high density fat and calories. You can get pretty full on grilled salmon or chicken over greens with a geggie side and a baked potato. Try baking sweet potatoes, they are so rich in nutrients and taste sweet and fantastic with cinnamon sprinkled on top mixed with a few drops of water. Potatoes are so satisfying, which is why I often prefer them over rice. If you love lemon, marinate your chicken in lemon for a few hours before grilling or baking it. It gives off such a delightful aroma and, better yet, it makes the fish or chicken taste fantastic, especially when served with steamed brown rice with pineapple. The taste is indescribably delicious.

There are so many wonderful foods out there that don't have high calories. You just have to take the time to try them. It may take a period of adjustment, especially if you are so used to cooking in lots of olive oil and butter, but you too can eventually adapt. Besides, just think what that change alone will do to your weight and see if it still isn't enough to get you started.

Cooking for small children can definitely be a challenge. Unfortunately, children can take longer to acquire a taste for veggies or lightly seasoned meals. They usually prefer mashed potatoes, french fries, and that's okay, but just watch the salt and oil or butter content. When making them mashed potatoes, try using light butter and skim milk instead. It tastes the same, and in fact, your husband probably won't notice either. With him, you can add a little garlic powder and some other herbs, and he'll love it.

If you are having friends over for dinner or meeting them at a restaurant and you are worried about eating too much, have a huge glass of iced water first. In fact, anytime you sit down to eat, drink a large glass of cold water, even if you aren't thirsty. That actually tricks your body into thinking you are full, and you'll find you won't eat nearly as much.

Another good idea is, before you eat dinner, have a protein shake and if you don't want to take the time to make one, you can buy a small plastic shaker with protein powder in it. Just add cold water and you will be full in seconds. Although it gives you additional protein and takes away your appetite, it is low enough in calories (about ninety calories per serving) that it shouldn't be an issue. I often do that when I go out and I would usually say, "I'm just not very hungry today," and that shuts people up. The good news is you'll probably get up the next morning a pound lighter.

If you feel you have to have a cocktail (just because everyone else is having one), watch what you drink. A margarita has approximately 500 calories, a mojito has 150 and is more satisfying to your palate. Instead of a rum and coke, which has 350 calories, have a rum with diet coke, which only has 150 calories. Instead of a glass of wine at 400 calories, have a wine spritzer with soda water at 120 calories. And the really great news is that the next morning, you can actually expect to not have any hangover.

So you see, there are indeed so many ways to enjoy eating without having to miss out on your favorite foods or dining out.

> "Blessed are those who hunger and thirst for they are sticking to their diets."—Author unknown, 50 years ago

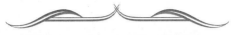

Fitness Tidbits

Morning workouts tend to be better at burning fat, whereas afternoon and evening workouts tend to be better for strength and endurance training. And if you have any heart issues, there is far less risk in the late afternoon.

Being physically fit refers to cardiovascular fitness—that is, your excellent usage of oxygen within the lungs and heart while you exercise. If you are fit according to medical standards, you will not easily get winded walking at least a mile, and it should take no more than twenty minutes if you walk briskly.

To increase fat loss, intermingle your routine—whatever it might be—and mix slow movements such as walking and jogging with fast ones. For instance, I do what I call a "walk-jog" for an average of four miles almost daily as one of my fitness routines. I walk briskly for fifteen minutes, then jog for fifteen minutes and on and on. Whatever is your exercise of choice—walking, jogging, swimming, biking, or using the treadmill in a gym—it becomes an outstanding fat-burning technique in no time. Try it and you'll be pleased with the results.

When you do aerobic exercise, the muscles demand a constant supply of oxygen, which in turn, benefit the heart, lungs, and your body in general. However, anaerobic exercise will increase your strength because the muscles don't depend on the oxygen. Anaerobic exercise is definitely less stressful, but the benefits are outstanding. You develop lean muscle, excellent muscle tone, endurance, and greater strength. A mixture of both is the ideal, aerobic and anaerobic.

It doesn't matter really if you eat during the day or evening. Your body won't burn any more or less fat, sugar, or calories in general. We often hear it does make a difference, but honestly, it doesn't. Going to bed full, however, will affect your quality of sleep, and it isn't good for the digestive tract. You might be restless rather than relaxed.

Personally, I always wanted something sweet in late evening, especially ice cream or frozen yogurt. Since I have a history of migraine headaches, I've cut out most of the triggers that set off the headache attacks, but I refuse to cut out the ice cream. Finally, after years of nightly headaches, I gave up my indulgence for ice cream and just allow it once in a while. When a particular food causes a great deal of pain or discomfort, you soon learn to avoid that food, no matter how much you love it.

> "If you don't allow time for exercise, be prepared to spend a great deal of time being ill."—Author unknown

I'm Starving, Let's Eat

A few years ago, I read a most interesting book by Kevin Trudeau, "natural cures", that is "natural cures they don't want you to know about." The sad but true fact is that we do live in not just a fast food diet society but a fast-everything society, as far as I'm concerned. Our lives have become so hectic and stressful in spite of the so-called time-saving devices that are supposed to make our lives more comfortable, with many of us working long hours and oftentimes on overtime just to earn a few extra dollars. With raising children, maintaining and cleaning a household, cooking, attending meetings, children events, volunteering, plus countless other things in our daily routine, we just don't have enough time to squeeze everything in. Who has time to prepare meals, let alone trying to get everyone to the table at the same time.to think about healthy meals is just added stress, when it's much easier, perhaps a little costlier to pick up and take home. "thanks kentucky colonel and pizza places!

Back to *Natural Cures*. I do agree with the fact that we are what we eat, plain and simple. What is amazing is, if you choose to have two cups of coffee in the morning and consider that as breakfast (because you don't want to be late for work, so you quickly go to the drive-through window at McDonald's because that is on the way), then so be it. Then lunchtime rolls around and you didn't bring lunch. Again, you go for the fast meal for a substitute and, of course you take the coke and chips along with that. And once again on your way home from work, kentucky colonel happens to be right down the street, so bingo! Then during the little time you might have to enjoy watching TV, you want something sweet. You might feel full, have some indigestion or gas, but as far as you're concerned, there's nothing major. You tell yourself you still look good and just pleasingly plump, even though you're now twenty pounds overweight.

Honestly though, if you could see what happens internally after months and years of eating this kind of food, it might scare you enough to keep you from ever eating again. Excessive fatty tissues surround your organs, and arterial walls thicken which, makes it difficult for the blood to flow smoothly. These are just the basic problems, but believe me, there are many more.

A man did a supervised study by living only on hamburgers and fries for thirty days, and the result: he gained over twenty pounds, became very tired, sleepy, and lethargic. He developed headaches, upset stomach, constipation and diarrhea. To make matters worse, his blood pressure and cholesterol spiraled out of control.

For you fried food lovers out there, eat fried food sparingly. It is by far the most dangerous thing that you can eat and will do the most harm to your body. Stop saying, "Fried food tastes great," because when you really try to savor it you only get that greasy aftertaste, and it makes your breath smell not so pleasant too!

Earlier on, I've also said that you can lose weight on just about any kind of food as long as you take in less than what your body can burn off, and it is true. But think about what it is doing to you internally when you eat unhealthy foods.

When you have a few minutes, try looking up images of people who live on fatty foods and those who get by with whole grains and non-fatty foods. If you can handle the images, now try to see what excessive fat looks like internally—the liver, heart, and kidneys, among others. Sometimes on TV, disclaimers would usually say, "Images are very graphic and might be difficult to watch." That's how shocking to look at the images often are, and all because of what you eat. The illnesses that can occur because of obesity are overshadowed in any case by the shortened lifespan if you continue eating foods that just aren't doing you any good day in and day out.

"Life is a journey, enjoy the ride."—Billy Graham

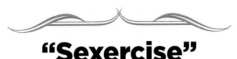

"Sexercise"

Got your attention, didn't it? Here are a few "unique" ways to not only burn more calories but enjoy the process! While making love when you are on your back and your legs are up in the air slowly lower them, then raise them, first with straight legs then bend at the knees. You'll not only get a flatter tummy but your partner will think you are really excited since he or she can really feel the difference. Of course, you can't tell your partner what you are doing and why because that will seriously demasculinate him immediately!

There is no better way to lose approximately 350 calories an hour. Next time your partner feels amorous, and you don't because you had a long frustrating day at work, or there were problems with the kids, and you didn't have time to exercise, you just want to go to bed and sleep, think again! You might even end up a pound thinner.

Here is a general list of calories burned during "Sexercise."—Author unknown

Male ready: zero calories
Female not quite ready: 275 calories

Normal position: Male 300 calories
Normal position: Female 150 calories
Recovery: Male: Going to the kitchen, could be a negative 350 calories
Recovery Female: Going to the bathroom,10 calories.

Moral of the story...the more you move, the more you lose!

"A bear however hard he tries grows tubby without exercise."—Author A.A.Milne

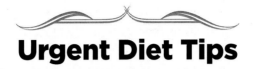

Urgent Diet Tips

Always eat some protein for breakfast and ideally, a small amount of complex carbohyadrates. For breakfast, you can have oatmeal with a little fruit and skim milk, eggs, slice of toast, or even a protein shake in a can, or a protein bar if you really are in a hurry. What's important is that you eat something. What you don't realize when you skip breakfast is that your blood sugar will be out of whack, and you'll tend to grab something fattening, which does absolutely nothing to you but make you more ravenous later on. What is great about protein is that it breaks down slowly, giving you a feeling of satisfaction for a while longer, and you tend to not eat as much junk food for the day.

Eat fresh fruits and vegetables over juice whenever you can. The fresh natural form has enzymes in them to keep your immune system at its peak of performance. Also, the fresh fruit and vegetables have lots of fiber, which give you the sensation of fullness for a longer period of time than juices alone do. I understand time sometimes is the issue, that you don't have time to stand there and peel fruit. Luckily, the stores now have fruits and veggies already pared and sliced and wrapped for freshness. These are great in a pinch, just as the small cans of V8, and I do use them from time to time. But the key is to do this sparingly.

Always have protein and a piece of fruit between meals. This is a great habit to get into because you will want to eat far less at mealtime. There are so many wonderful protein snacks, shakes, and bars now that make it really easy to get your protein in. You do have to be careful, however, because many of the bars are much higher in fat content, and you don't typically take in over fifteen to twenty grams of fat a day. Ideally, to lose a fair amount of weight rather quickly, cut out as much fat as possible. I personally find that fat calories are far more difficult to burn off than carbohydrate calories. Hopefully, you know your body well enough to know what works best for you.

Eat red meat as seldom as possible. Yes, red meat contains lots of protein, which is a good thing, but again, even the leanest of meats have at least eleven grams of fat in a 4.5-ounce portion. It's usually the saturated fat and cholesterol in the meat that are the culprits and work against us. "chick-fils" has the greatest AD campaign showing a group of cows with signs around their necks that say, "Eat chicken." How true that is. Lean red meat is okay once in a while, but in addition to the high fat content in even the leanest of meats, it has a tendency of making you bloated and sluggish. Just keep that in mind if you tend to be a big meat-eater. One tablespoon of olive oil in balsamic vinegar makes a great zesty dressing, but just don't overdo it. You want the dressing to enable you to enjoy the greens in the salad. We are fortunate today because there are so many light dressings such as Kens Raspberry Vinaigrette that are absolutely packed with flavor and without the fat.

Have a glass of wine if you like but don't use one of those huge wine goblets; use the four-ounce ones instead. Learn to sip it and enjoy the aroma and savor the taste. Wine, like anything else you put into your body, will turn into fat, so moderation is always the key. Since I'm not a fan of wine, I actually put ice into my wine. If you can drink champagne, have that over wine instead. It doesn't take much champagne at all to feel relaxed.

Do not weight in daily. It can steer you off course if you find out you haven't lost a pound that day. At that point, you just might want to say, "The heck with it. Since I didn't lose a pound today, I might as well eat what I want and start again tomorrow." This is the wrong attitude. So many variables—menstrual cycle, constipation, water retention, extra salt that you might have had in your food the day before—enter into the picture when you weigh on a daily basis. Medications you are on can make a huge difference since they often make you lethargic and bloated. Oftentimes when you ignore that, you drop an additional pound the next day. If you didn't lose a pound that day or any day, walk around in a shopping center if it is too warm out, go for a swim, go to the gym, or just do something physical rather than go off your diet when you feel discouraged go for a quick walk. I guarantee you by the next weigh-in you will have lost the double amount of weight.

One more tip: If you didn't lose much weight and you thought you were doing everything right, don't eat anything with salt for two days, not even the chicken breasts you just bought from the meat department, or the cheese you wanted to sample. There is so much sodium in everything we eat that we don't realize we are getting far more than the one teaspoon our bodies need. Also, keep in mind that your body retains two pounds of weight for every teaspoon you eat. If you eat everything that does not have sodium in it, you will be amazed at how much you can lose. The bulk of your food will most likely be fresh fruits and vegetables and fresh fish. Try this, and you will have a really quick weight loss.

"If the t.v. and the refrigerator weren't so far apart, some people would never get any exercise!"—Joey Adams

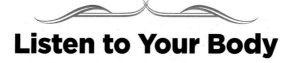

Listen to Your Body

We all pretty much know what to eat because it is drilled into us everywhere on TV, news, shows like *Dr. Oz*, *Oprah*, and the *Biggest Loser*. Little fat or low fat, healthy fat, little or no sugar, definitely no corn syrup, high protein, preferrably chicken, fish, and some red meat—these about say it all. I do basically follow choices; however, I firmly believe that when you exercise approximately an hour a day and go about your daily living activities with a certain amount of zest, you can eat a diet balanced with carbohydrates, protein, and some fat.

Take for instance my basic daily diet: I start the day with a yogurt and an orange, go play tennis or walk briskly with jogging spurts for an hour and a half or two hours (if time allows it), and then have a glass of skim milk and a bagel with cream cheese and jam or lox (whichever is on sale).;On my way to work a few hours later, I would have a grilled chicken snack wrap often, and for dinnertime I would have a small piece of fish, veggies, brown rice, or sushi, which was a staple of mine while living all those years in Hawaii. And when I get home at night, I'd top it off with a large double scoop of cookies-and-cream ice cream and three cookies. The good news is, once you've reached your weight goal, you can eat as I do. In fact, by increasing my exercise time, I still lose weight eating this way.

I don't measure my food; I definitely don't starve. I often use light dressing over fat-free, sometimes even regular, dressing like chunky blue cheese, which is my favorite. I do prefer light mayonnaise to regular mayonnaise (regular tastes too greasy to me), and I do eat Brummel & Brown butter instead of the regular one. I prefer skim milk and do away from gravy and creamy sauces. My food choices help me to stay slim mainly because I don't like fatty or oily-tasting things. I don't like fried foods and am also not a lover of lots of Italian or French dishes. The point is, there are no great magical tricks or mysterious secrets to losing weight, but one way to get there is by listening to your body, and by that I mean how your digestive tract responds to certain foods that you take in. Here is an example using my digestive system: In my case, fatty and spicy foods give diarrhea and make me feel bloated and gaseous. I don't like staying up at night with these abdominal problems and have learned to listen to my body. It has taken me years to accept the fact that I can't tolerate most Chinese food, and it triggers migraine headaches on me as most alcoholic beverages do (one reason I rarely drink). On the other hand, my downfall has always been dessert. Oftentimes, I'd rather walk or jog an extra three miles just so I can eat ice cream. I had a friend in Hawaii whose family owned an inexpensive Chinese restaurant. Often I would go and watch them prepare some of the dishes that I just mentioned and if you ever saw it made you wouldn't eat it either. The steamed chicken dishes in veggies, and similar dishes are fine however.there are many things we seem to like such as sausage, hot dogs, imitation crab as several examples. However, since we are not the chef and are unsure of the spices and seasonings used in preparation certain dishes even though smell terrific may not agree with us.

The bottom line, you should know what you can eat, what agrees with you and what doesn't; whether the food items are good for you or not is another issue entirely. What is really good for you isn't usually what you want to eat, but the good news is you can change. You can learn to have better, healthier eating habits, and feel better from the inside out.

What's nice with my lifestyle is that since I enjoy exercise so much (because I look at it not as exercise but my playtime), I can have pancakes once in a while smothered in syrup and don't feel the least bit guilty about it. I have to admit though, I have been living this way for so long, and because I do have a nutritional background, I know approximately how many calories, fat and sugar grams, and protein are in everything that I eat. I know when I go overboard and when I'm on track. My mind just automatically keeps track of every calorie that goes into my mouth. I know when I have to cut back and when I can eat more.

You too can get to that state. It does take work and commitment, but the reward is so wonderful—you feel and look absolutely fantastic! You might as well accept the fact that each and every one of us has to exercise and move it to lose it, because like it or not, thin or fat, it is what your body requires. None of us want the health problems caused by excessive eating and inactive lifestyles as we get older.

> "I never worry about diets. The only carrots that interest me are the number you get in a diamond."
> —Mae West

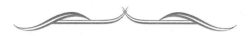

What Does Fitness Really Mean?

When you hear the word "fitness," I'm sure you immediately visualize a pretty lady in workout shorts and sports bra happily jogging down the street. Actually, it encompasses several aspects such as stretching, aerobic and anaerobic activities, and healthy eating habits.

Stretching is vital whether you work out or not. Typically, you should do a full body stretch as soon as you wake up in the morning. It can actually kick-start your day. Try to observe a cat. A cat will nap on and off for about eighteen hours every day. Every time it wakes up from its nap, it will stretch out its entire body. I always marvel at watching my cat. She'll stretch for thirty seconds then go right back to sleep. I never have been able to adopt great sleep habits, but I do stretch a lot, even at work in my office after sitting at the computer for an hour or more. Stretching definitely keeps you limber. As people get older, their joints tend to become stiff and sore upon movement, and this can be alleviated to a great extent simply by stretching a few minutes daily, no matter what age. It will improve your balance and coordination and will prevent most of the back pain people seem to develop over the years because it strengthens all the muscles from the neck down to the ankles. It also improves circulation, which helps to lower blood pressure, so as you see, if you can include a five- or ten-minute stretching routine throughout your day, your body will definitely thank you.

Often you hear people talking about the core muscles, especially orthopedic surgeons, chiropractors, and personal trainers. Core muscles are the muscle groups that make up the abs, back, and pelvis. If you've ever done a routine at a gym, you've probably included Circuit training. This series helps strengthen all the core muscles or central body as well as every other part of your body. Depending on your problematic areas, you might spend more time on one group of muscles over another. I can speak for most women and we tend to do a lot of abdominal work, thinking this will help flatten our tummy. Unfortunately, you really have to do a lot more than that, and I mean a lot of reps to make a difference on the abs. The circuit routine consists of resistance exercises with different weight levels from ten pounds up to two hundred. Typically, women stay within a ten-pound to a thirty-five-pound range depending on which muscle group they are working on. When working the abdomenal machine, many women can handle a higher weight resistant level. I don't recommend higher weights on the leg-raise machine because you can easily injure yourself in that. In a circuit, you want to add weight little by little as your body adapts to each level comfortably.

One of the biggest problems I've seen at a gym is when a person starts a routine at a higher weight level than he or she can handle. I think sometimes pride gets in the way, especially if it is a man trying to impress his female trainer or an attractive female in the gym. As a result, the next day he'll be so sore that he'll lay off going back to the gym for a few days. Unfortunately, he'll do the same thing all over again because he'll feel he can. Anytime you use a group of muscles more than you usually do, it will hurt! But the pain goes away, and you will survive. More often than not, however, the person gives up entirely and tells his friends that gyms are a waste of time. The thing is, when you only follow the regimen correctly, it will certainly pay off. Your overweight body will eventually take on a healthy lean look.

Oftentimes, women have the opposite problem. They tend to give up easily for several reasons:

1. They don't set the starter weight high enough for fear of getting sore. If the weights are set too low, you don't accomplish anything. Your strength can only improve by training your muscles to work a little harder each time. You do need to exert a little more effort to be successful just like in every other aspect of life.

2. When some women feel stiff and sore, they sometimes give up for fear of "bulking up" and getting too muscular. I hear that so often, and some are so stubborn about it they don't want to accept the truth that it generally takes hours and hours in the gym daily and hundreds of reps to create more muscle. The level that most of us work out at will not make you bulky or excessively muscular. Look at female bodybuilders. I have a

close friend who lives in Maui and who is a partial bodybuilder. She won't get involved in any other sport but spends four hours a day at the gym to get that muscular definition. She feels that's what makes a woman beautiful.

3. Sometimes, women say, "I can't lose weight when I work out at a gym. I always gain weight." That is true, sometimes a person will gain weight not from working out but typically from eating more. I'm very guilty of that. Too often I cheat, thinking I've justified eating a big lunch or dinner, since I did an extra hard workout that day. Sure, you burn a lot more calories in a day, perhaps up to six hundred, but it doesn't mean you can order everything on the menu! A person has to run an additional six miles to burn six hundred calories. If we are honest with ourselves, we rarely do that, but we still like to eat as though we ran six miles. Just imagine how fast you would lose weight if you stick to a fairly strict diet and work out hard. You can drop fifteen pounds in a month easily. You will go to bed starving, but you'll look great in the morning. When you feel ravenous after a gym workout, drink lots of water, then head to the nearest produce store and eat a water-based fruit like melons or strawberries. That will hold you until you get home or to a restaurant. Staying really hydrated is a wonderful way to trick your growling stomach (for a few minutes, anyway) into thinking you aren't that hungry and can wait another hour to eat lunch.

4. Sometimes, people give up because it can be difficult sticking to a routine. It's much easier to go home after work when you've had a difficult day, or there was a lot of traffic that's taking you an extra half hour to get home. It does take a fierce determination and perseverance, which is one reason why two-thirds of society is overweight. After doing this for thirty plus years, I feel worse if I don't physically work out every day. In fact, I've often driven a few friends crazy because I insist on exercise daily, even when on vacation. As a result, not too many people offer to go on vacation with me!

Having a lot of strength and flexibility essentially helps you get through every activity you want to get involved in. An outstanding benefit is that it prevents injuries from happening. When someone gets a back or knee injury, oftentimes he does gain weight because he can't do his normal exercise routine and still eats as though he can. Unfortunately, it has a way of compounding itself, so the moral of the story is to try to not get any injuries. Over the years, the only kinds of injuries I've gotten are "overuse" injuries.

Once your body adapts to a routine, it does become comfortable, and you feel as though you can go on for hours, which I have done and paid the price for. I used to jog about six to ten miles daily, and a few times ended up with bilateral stress fractures. These are very small stress fractures that look like twigs on a tree, but they can really cause a lot of pain. I've found the best way to overcome them is to tenderly work through them without stopping altogether. Once you stop for a while, you have to build up your endurance all over again. You can do some wonderful strength training exercises at home on the floor or on a mat. If you are doing an abdominal routine, remember to always hold your stomach in throughout the workout. This actually tightens the abdominal muscles, which is what you're striving for in the first place. There are many books out there and a plethora of websites on strengthening the core muscles.

Let's get back to what fitness really means. As discussed, one aspect is stretching, another is the resistance training to increase strength and endurance. Endurance means the length of time you can walk, jog, climb, dance, etc. without getting tired and out of breath. Getting out of breath upon exertion is not a good thing, and some people blame it on age, while others blame it on working too many hours, but frankly it means you are overweight 95% of the time. Of course, there are those who have bona fide respiratory conditions or cardiac conditions that will tire you out, so those are excusable. For the rest of us, there are no excuses. I've even worked with a number of men and women who are relatively slender, yet get tired very easily. Typically, it means they haven't done any strength training, which everyone does need no matter what size or shape. This can happen with a twelve-hour workday, which many people are doing now, so they are limited on time to learn to get stronger. Some of these people don't have much of an appetite, while others would rather drink their calories. If I'm going to have extra calories, I would want it to taste great.

For an older lady, I'm so proud that I have excellent endurance. Often, I compete with people half my age in singles tennis, men and women, and I easily outlast them. I've indeed been accused of being the Energizer Bunny's mother! I used to play singles tennis twice a week with a man half my age. Looking at him, you would think he was in great shape. He also went through college on a tennis scholarship. The sad thing was he had to sit down every fifteen minutes or so to rest for a few minutes. I'd keep practicing while he rested., and he'd say, "Who are you really, Carol? Don't you ever get tired?" We played in the Hawaiian heat and still it never bothered me. Now living in Florida, the heat and humidity no longer bother me at all, thank goodness. I really feel blessed as I see others often sweltering in the heat.

A few years ago, I worked with a twenty-six-year old woman who needed to lose twenty-five-plus pounds, and I told her I could help her lose the weight, but that she had to commit to doing everything I would show her as far as physical activity goes. She said, "No problem, I'm young and relatively in good shape." If you've been to the Hawaiian islands, particularly in Maui, you'd know that there are many steep hills and mountains throughout Hawaii. As a challenge, I would try to jog up at least one steep hill twice a week to help keep up my endurance level. The hills averaged at least a mile up.

On the first training day, I worked with this young woman, and she was jogging in place at ground level, raring to go. I told her we would only go up about a third of the way the first day, and she quickly said, "No problem." We were about halfway up to the stopping point, and I noticed she was out of breath, her face a dark shade of red, and she just stopped. She refused to go any further and just sat there in the middle of the sidewalk. I told her she could do it, and that she should just take it as slow as she needed to go. She got mad and said she hated me. I was a mean trainer, but she reluctantly trudged onward and made it, at least up to the point we wanted to reach.

Yes, it is hard to start a routine, especially when there are stairs and hills involved, but there is no better way to build that endurance level than hills as far as I'm concerned. If you live in a flat area, get a stair stepper. They are outstanding for your butt and thighs as well. Each time we got together, which was about three times a week depending on schedules, we built up her time and distance little by little. At 3 months I was so proud of her. She lost thirty-five pounds, and her body developed this long lean look. Her legs that were always skinny became shapely. We dressed up one night to go out and celebrate, and it was such an emotional experience because she said, "Carol, thanks to you for pushing me and believing I could do it. I feel beautiful for the first time in my life."

Once you commit to getting into shape, the rewards are tenfold. You not only do feel beautiful, but you gain confidence that you've only dreamed about. We really can be all that we want to be; only it takes a lot of faith, commitment, and determination.

> "I don't know why gyms have so many mirrors.
> I know what I look like, that's why I'm here."
> —Author unknown

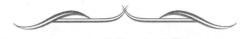

I'm Just Not Hungry

You may say, why is this in a book about diet and exercise? Unfortunately, how we feel often dictates when and what we eat or don't eat. For that matter, not eating is as bad for your body as overeating. For years, we've heard about the harmful effects of anorexia and bulimia. There still is a big problem with women in the entertainment and modeling field in relation to eating habits. These young women are so afraid of gaining weight that they literally starve themselves until they have no fat on their bodies at all. There are three types of body fat: first is the structural fat, which is necessary to give support to the organs and smooth contour to the body; second is the normal fat, which is what gives you energy; and the last is the exogenous or abnormal fat, which is the unsightly and dangerous type of fat. Women seem to gain this from their waist down, and men are more likely to gain this in their abdomen.

Obviously, the only fat you want to lose is the abnormal fat. Everyone absolutely has to have structural and normal fat to survive and to be healthy. When you starve, your body loses the good fat. You become very weak, to say the least, and you are subject to a host of illnesses, which can lead to organ failure or worse, heart failure and death. What is really sad is that these people, primarily women, think they look beautiful. They look at the least amount of fat as being ugly. When they get to this point, there are serious emotional and mental issues. From time to time, some of the prime time talk shows interview some of these women, particularly actresses, because they are the ones in the limelight and whom we have name recognition with. Often, they are ill more than healthy and end up missing a lot of work. My nephew, Johnny Pacar, is an actor in Hollywood. He told me when you are in front of a camera, you appear to be heavier than you really are, and that is why actors in general are so obsessed about their weight. It can mean getting a part or not. He too watches his weight but does eat healthy foods rather than a lot of junk food.

High fashion models, for some reason, are usually very thin and tall. They aren't born thin but have learned not to eat for fear of gaining unsightly fat. While I was in college, I did some modeling for a high-end department store one semester just so I could get some free outfits. I loved always being one of the best dressed women on campus. In fact, I always worked two jobs while in school to be able to buy great outfits to wear on campus, aside from helping pay for my education. I had so much fun doing it but knew I wasn't built to make a career out of it. When asked about it at a banquet the store put on for us after the fashion show season, I said I could never be a model just because I was shorter than most but because I really loved to eat. Everyone chuckled except another woman, who was also a model in those shows. She said, "Honestly, Carol, do you always have to say something ridiculous?" and I replied, "It's not ridiculous to love to eat!"

Which leads me to the next issue: how much is "too much"? I like feeling happy, and food definitely makes me feel happy, if only for a moment. Unfortunately, most of us go beyond happy or sad and use food as a crutch. It becomes our comfort in a stress-filled world. In the case of actresses and models, fear of getting fat becomes the crutch so they don't eat, and that is just as dangerous. Most of us recognize those times in our lives when we can't eat, but these are just momentary in the grand scheme of things. Typically, these are brought on by stress and anxiety, but there is a difference since they are usually short-term.

Some instances in your daily life may bring a momentary loss of hunger, and it could perhaps be because you had a bad day at work and your boss had put some ridiculous pressure on you to perform a task that you just couldn't complete by the end of the day. He was upset, which made you feel stupid and incompetent, and you leave an hour and a half later than you normally do. Then you rush out the door, cussing as only you know how, and when you get home, the first thing that comes out of your family's mouth is, "You are late. When can we eat?" And you think, *Can't my family ever think about me instead of them all the time?* Then you turn to your husband and say, "Couldn't you have made dinner for a change? Do I have to do everything around here as you slam pots and pans on the stove?" And by the time dinner is ready, you simply can't eat.

I had a similar experience a few years ago while living in Maui. My company had sent over from Honolulu a corporate person to train my staff on a new computer program. I'm friendly, outgoing, intelligent, but definitely not great on administrative procedures and especially on new procedures on the computer. We should have learned the program in a few hours, but needless to say, it took me a few hours longer to grasp the technique. By that time, the trainer was so upset with me that we had a very unpleasant exchange. She said, "I even voted for you, Carol, to be the employee of the year of all the stores." She then abruptly left after saying I was impossible to work with. I was upset but shocked that I was even being considered for employee of the year and thought that little argument just ruined my chances for the award. By the time I drove across the island back to my home in Lahaina, my boyfriend said, "What took you so long?" That of course made me even more upset as I slapped some food on the table. I just couldn't eat nor speak to him. He didn't even do anything wrong! How often we lash out at others when everything could have been avoided in the first place. The good news though is that the next morning I had dropped three pounds. The bad news is I had an upset boyfriend, which was really my fault.

I really don't recommend losing weight that way. You may think you have won the battle, but you're actually losing the war. In my case, I did, however, call the trainer and apologize profusely. She did go on to vote for me, and I did win the Employee of the Year award in spite of it, much to my surprise. I was so shocked when they called my name out to step forward out of over 100 employees that I truly was speechless. There are times in our life that we just can't eat! Even in the great times, however.

On a side note, starvation diets, whether they be from an actual diet to lose weight or from an emotional upset, the side effects can be horrendous. Initially, you get a violent headache that doesn't go away for hours, sometimes days. In addition, you get lightheaded, dizzy, and nauseated; some people actually start shaking. If these are the physical symptoms you feel, just imagine what is going on internally that you aren't aware of yet. Your body goes into ketosis, which causes extremely bad breath. You become so weak that it is an effort to do even the simplest of tasks. You become so irritable that no one wants to be around you, and imagine compounding that with bad breath! Your immune system can virtually shut down if you go into a strict diet, 500 calories or less. This leaves you susceptible to colds, flu, and goodness knows what else. You have to be smart about your food intake. There is a fine line between what is healthy and what isn't.

> "The toughest part of a diet isn't watching what you eat but watching what everyone else eats."—Author unknown

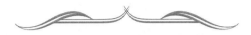

The More You Move, the More You Burn

You might think, that's a stupid comment, everyone knows that, but here are some alarming facts you don't know about. If you have a sedentary job and work a normal eight-hour workday, and if you sit at least six hours a day, your metabolism drops approximately up to a rate of 35%. Your body will burn approximately one calorie per minute instead of the normal three calories per minute for a person who is fairly active. Add one to two hours of aerobic exercise a day, and your metabolism skyrockets and your body continues to burn a higher rate of calories long after you are through with your exercise regimen.

Now, I know many of you have a hard time coming up with an extra hour a day to do an aerobic exercise routine, but here are some helpful tips on how to rev up your metabolism so that your body will increase the number of calories it burns in a day.

1. Eat more protein. By replacing some of your carbs or fat with protein, your body works less harder in digesting them that it usually does with protein, hence increasing your metabolic rate.

2. Eat more often. If you eat something every few hours rather than waiting six or seven hours between meals, your metabolic rate increases, in part due to digesting the foods even something as simple as an orange.

3. Energy drinks definitely can rev up your metabolism, but stay clear of the high sugar and high calorie drinks. Those with caffeine and taurine are very effective; the caffeine gets your heart rate going, while the taurine, which is an amino acid, helps burn fat. Just be careful you don't get too jittery or nervous and don't drink these before bedtime, or you might have a problem sleeping.

4. Double your water intake. Studies indicate that those who drink eight glasses or more of water a day also double their calorie burn.

5. Eat lots of water-based fruits and vegetables. These will give you the sensation of fullness, especially between meals.

6. Build more muscle. Do some resistance exercises. If you don't belong to a gym, use a 1-pound can of anything in each hand and start raising and lowering your arms 12 times. Ten seconds later, do another set of 12 reps. Every pound of muscle burns 6 calories an hour just to sustain itself, whereas each pound of fat burns only 2 calories an hour.

7. Alter your work out regimen. If you tend to walk briskly, jog for 5 minutes, then resume walking. If you prefer bike riding, get off your bike for 5 minutes and walk your bike. Every time you suddenly do a change then resume your normal routine, it revs up your metabolic rate.

In general, the biggest health hazard is sitting for hours on end, even if you are fit. As soon as you get into a sedentary mode, your metabolism comes to a complete halt. Here are some tips to get moving without going to the gym.

1. When putting laundry away, don't grab the whole pile. Instead, put up one towel at a time, one shirt, and so on and so forth.
2. Cook with heavy pots and pans. The heavier they are, the harder to lift, hence your body works harder with this simple task.
3. When cooking, instead of mixing with a blender, do it by hand. Your arm muscles will thank you for it a month later.
4. During TV commercials, stand up and march in place.
5. When traveling, book a hotel room on a higher floor and walk up instead of using the elevator; same with the office. If your office is on the second or third floor, take the stairs. Stairs will do wonders to your backside and abs, believe it or not.

6. When waiting for a flight, instead of sitting there and staring into space, take a walk. Besides, you'll be sitting long enough on the plane.

7. Don't take the people movers in the terminal, unless you're late, of course. Walk the walk!

8. If driving on a road trip, get out of the car and walk around every hour or so. Don't try to save an hour by going as long as you can without stopping. I have to say, that tends to be a favorite of men! Notice their belly. I'd be willing to bet they can use the brief walk break too!

9. Regarding errands, definitely park further from the store, or walk through the whole store once then go to the specific departments that you are looking for.

10. Stop shopping online. The store will love you, and so will your hips!

11. Do a few arm raises with your shopping bags. I personally love doing this one. It's a given.

12. For fun, go for a hike, or a romantic walk in the woods.

13. Go to an art museum or to a zoo if you love animals.

14. Rent a kayak; it's great for the upper arms and just being out in the water is relaxing too.

15. If you love being around water, you can also go to a restaurant at a marina other than go swimming or beach walking. It is always fun to walk around the boats.

16. When at home in the bedroom, give your mate a massage. It may sometimes be a hard work, but

your hands and arms will look great after a few of these sessions.

17. Years ago, there was an article in Ladies' Home Journal that was entitled, "Instead of a Plate, Reach for Your Mate." You would be astounded how many calories and exercise you get if you do exactly this.

18. When you want to talk over your day with your husband, do so while taking a walk.

19. Move your cell phone out of reach at home after work so that you have to run for it when it rings.

20. On a weekend, rake the leaves, mow the lawn, work in the yard. It feels great doing these in the autumn air.

21. If you have a dog, don't take him to the groomer; give him a bath yourself. It can be very amusing as well as a good exercise session.

Hopefully, you've enjoyed some, if not all, of the tips listed above. Indeed, these will help raise your metabolic level so that you will burn more as you move it to lose it. After all, going to the gym isn't always what makes the difference.

> "Exercise is done against one's wishes and maintained only because the alternative is worse."
> —George Sheehan

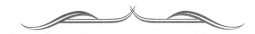

Stress versus De-stress

Stress: pressure or tension exerted on a material object; the body's reaction to changes that require a physical, mental, or emotional adjustment. One of several definitions in the Merrill Webster dictionary.

One of the most common reasons clients state for gaining weight and not exercising is stress. If you are living a normal life—looking after a spouse or mate, family, work, children's school and activities, deadlines at work, events and personal activities to attend to, to name a few—most likely you'll claim the same. It is a significant part of life, and you can't get away from it no matter what. Just getting to work on time in the heavy traffic can particularly set off your day, especially if you are already a few minutes late. And if you have children who are still at school and have to get them to a bus stop by a specific time, it can certainly be stressful. Deciding what to make for dinner, let alone preparing it, can also be stressful. Even on holidays, often you feel a lot more stress than pleasure, which is sad. You lose sight of what holidays actually are about.

Stress affects your eating habits more than any other emotion. People often use it as an excuse, and I think that at that moment that person honestly feels that it's the stress he or she is going through that slows down his or her weight loss. I don't doubt that at all. In fact, it is proven that our bodies develop a higher amount of the hormone called cortisol when stressful. It actually is a corticosteroid that doesn't only cause you to want to eat more but also develops fatty deposits, making it more difficult to lose weight. I do feel, however, that since we can't get away from stress and how it affects our life, we can learn to counterbalance its negative effect. You have to learn how to control your response to stress rather than let stress take control of your response. You have to work through every other aspect of your life, thus, you need to learn to deal with stress. Many of you will say, "I don't know your particular situation that's causing you such anxiety," and that's true. But I do know there are different degrees of stress, and at some point it can cause considerable damage to us internally. It causes high blood pressure, diabetes, heart attacks, colitis, serious abdominal problems, and lack of sleep that can cause inability to concentrate, reason, and think.

I personally really react to stressful situations. I always hate it when someone says to me, "Relax, Carol, be cool." All the while I think to myself, "What do you mean relax? That person has no idea what I'm going through!" Stress will trigger a migraine attack so quickly on me that I can feel the headache come on before I have a chance to take the medication that aborts the headache. Next thing I know, I'm already suffering for hours.

So you see, I do understand how easy it is for someone to tell you to take it easy when you find it very difficult to do. In my case, the only good thing about the migraine is that once the headache occurs, I can't even think about food! Most people tend to eat a lot more—usually fattening foods—and they also usually eat more than what their bodies need, so they gain weight. They do that, thinking food will temporarily comfort them and make them forget about the stress. The next morning, however, when they get on the scale and see the weight gain, they realize they've only compounded the stressful problem. It becomes a vicious cycle that only gets worse. I remember one lady who once came into the weight loss clinic in tears. She was an emotional wreck because of stress, yet she became more stressed because I told her she had to give up certain foods for a while. She honestly felt that "healthy fats" such as nuts, olive oil, avocado, etc. wouldn't do her any harm, so I pointed out that too much of these "healthy fats" are equally harmful if you eat too much of them. This just made her more upset, and she automatically reached into her purse for a granola bar, then another.

Since we can't seem to live our lives without stress, we can instead learn to de-stress. The most effective way of de-stressing is exercise. At the very least, take a brief walk. When you're feeling so anxious you have to get out for a while, whatever you do, do not drive. Get out, walk around the building, or do jumping jacks, if that will help you. When those anxious feelings suddenly come over you, moving your body will definitely calm you down. When I was younger, every time I was stressed I would often blow up or yell at whoever was in my immediate area. That did nothing but hurt the friendship I had with those close to me. That's why it is best to go for a walk for a few minutes and allow yourself the time to calm down. When you feel calmer, your blood pressure and heart rate will also slow down. I always mention walking for a quick exercise but do whatever it takes in this case to calm down for exercise. Usually, stressful situations come on at work, so you better stick to walking, jogging in place, or going up and down some stairs if you happen to be working in a building with three stories or more. Any of these will help calm you down.

I don't recommend de-stressing with drugs or alcohol either because it does alter your thinking and your reaction time. Unfortunately, too many people have so many stressful days in their life that their first thought is, "I have to have a drink to calm down," or, "I need a couple of stiff drinks that will relax me. I had a really bad day at work, at home, with my husband, etc." Yes, alcohol will definitely relax you, cloud your thinking and your equilibrium among other things, and these are just a few more reasons why you shouldn't drive after drinking. I have been there and done that, so I do know firsthand what happens. I never want to go through that again. Sometimes, I look back at those years when I thought a few drinks after work would take care of most problems. How shortsighted I was, and young people the world over will continue to go through what I and millions of others have gone through. Had I known how much better I would have felt with a brisk walk or jogging instead of going to a bar, then I wouldn't have gone through what I had. Let alone the money that I would have saved.

I often hear the expression, "Life is for the young," and can't help but strongly disagree. I wish I had understood then what I know now about the negative effects alcohol has on the body versus the positive effects a great workout. I wonder if I would have been any different, but then I do believe people go through different phases in their life. Hopefully, you do grow out of those that have a negative effect on you.

When you suddenly feel stressed at work, or in a meeting, or even at home with a baby crying, a toddler screaming, as you are trying to juggle three things at once, you can't just drop everything and take a walk. I know at a time like that, there is nothing more that you would rather do than to disappear for a few minutes! I remember those feelings all too well. When it simply is impossible to get away, immediately try to put your mind at rest, close your eyes (not while you're holding a screaming baby, of course), and tell yourself, "This too shall pass. I can handle this. I can handle this." Just saying this a few times to myself has often put me into a calmer state, at least, until I had a chance to break away for a few minutes to clear my head.

Some people prefer to meditate for a few minutes when they are really stressed. This is another great thing to do to get your mind off the frustration you momentarily feel. Basically whatever you need to do that is good for your body when you feel the tension mounting, do it. As I stated earlier, you don't want to do anything that could harm you or others. And you really want to get your thoughts under control again, which is why a few minutes of exercise will do wonders for your psyche at these difficult times. The beauty of it is that you can lose weight, even during stressful times, and once you've figured out what works for you, you'll be in a weight loss mode because you won't let the negativity overtake you. You'll come out the winner and still feel like you can accomplish anything!

> "Eat, Sleep, and Swim. That's all I can do."
> —Michael Phelps, Olympic Gold Metalist

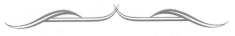

That Can't Be Me in That Mirror

L et's imagine for a moment it's Friday afternoon, the end of the work week. You've tried your best not to eat too much all week, knowing you'll be going out sometime over the weekend and partying a little. You've been pretty busy at work, so you didn't have time to really get in any exercise—which is nothing unusual for you— but you were on your feet a lot, running from one area to another, so that should have burned some calories, right? You and two of your girlfriends are going bike riding on Saturday, which is something you haven't done in years. You've decided to start a weekend exercise campaign, and bike riding is a great way to ease into it without getting completely exhausted. After all, you've only put on fifteen pounds in the last few months, and your boyfriend says you still look great, so what is the big deal? You'd rather get rid of this extra weight before it becomes twenty or twenty-five pounds though.

It's Saturday, lunchtime, and you've had a great workout with your friends after having ridden your bikes for about 8 miles. At least, you worked up a bit of a sweat, so you feel you deserve a terrific lunch. You all agree on your favorite Mexican restaurant because they serve the greatest stuffed burritos, chips, salsa, and guacamole. You actually pass on the drinks, since you are going out later with dates.

After lunch, you head to Macy's for its one-day Saturday sale because you get an extra 10% off only this Saturday! You decide to try on some great clothes, head for the dressing rooms, and scream as you attempt to try on your usual size 8. Then you swear someone changed these mirrors and put a cheaper version of mirrors in all the dressing rooms because your body couldn't possibly have those fatty areas! You never had those dimply thighs before. As you turn sideways and see the soft-rounded belly, you choke to hold back the tears that begin to flow, and you then blame it on the new birth control pills you're taking, somehow it just can't be your fault! Or you blame it on water weight.

Does this scenario sound familiar? It happens every day. Often we can't believe how we really do look, and until we go into a dressing room, that seems to be when reality hits. Dressing room comments can be funny though when you overhear them: "I look like a whale!"; "Look at this dress. I'm popping out all over just like the Pillsbury dough boy;" or better yet: "Why can't I find a print that makes me look twenty pounds lighter rather than twenty pounds heavier?" Someone could do a great comedy routine for a comedy show. Just from a woman's dressing room.

Did you ever notice that fitness centers always have mirrors that make you look really terrific and thin, whereas the dressing room mirrors make you look horrible? Shouldn't it be the other way around? I think both places would do a lot more business if that were the case. You'd feel like working out a lot harder if you looked heavier, perhaps even buying a better membership program with a personal trainer, just as you'd usually do when you're in a clothing store where you'd buy more clothes if you looked thinner in the mirror!

Did you ever notice that high-end restaurants always have strategically placed wonderful mirrors that seem to flatter every figure type? The owners want to sell food, and what better way than to have soft lighting and great mirrors that doesn't only show off the food perfectly but also the patrons. And there is usually a perfectly well-mannered, very charismatic maitre d'e, who immediately greets and flatters you, even before he seats you, knowing subtle phrases will lead to a generous tip.

Remember years ago where they had fun zones in amusement parks with distorted mirrors that made you look incredibly fat, and you'd laugh like crazy? Those days are long gone now. The good news is, no matter where you are, no matter what you see in the mirrors you look into, you can change what we see and be happy with it. It is entirely up to you how you want to change what you see. It really is how well you move it to lose it!

> "Our growing softness, our increasing lack of physical fitness, is a menace to our security."—John F. Kennedy

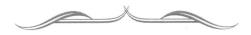

What Happened to Yesteryear's Athletes and Actors

Many of the rock-hard hot bodies of the '80s are the overweight, sagging, out-of–shape, soft bodies of 2013. What happened?

As Americans, we cherish athletes and top performers in most sports as well as highly paid actors and actresses. We seem to thrive on their lives and what happens to them over the years. That's actually one reason why I'm so grateful to not be in their shoes. Their lives are an open book in most cases, that they can't even enjoy a quiet dinner out, or take their children to the zoo without paparazzi everywhere snapping picture after picture of their every move.

Why are so many top athletes from years past now terribly out of shape? Football players, whether they were kickers or running backs are just as guilty as other top professional sports athletes, not just at the end of every season but even more so after they retire. The sad thing is they retire at a fairly young age, often in their late thirties or early forties because of all the wear and tear on their bodies and the fact that each year there are more of younger, tougher, and leaner players coming along who are better fit for the positions.

Take for instance, some of the basketball greats who are seven feet tall and 275 pounds but still have to watch what they eat now, even retired from basketball. They too find that even for them it's very easy to pack on the pounds, but that taking it off isn't as easy as it once was when they would train for hours at a time during season. Some previous baseball greats, in particular, are going through the same frustrating scenario as well as top golfers.

No matter what sports arena the pro athelete was in, with the extraordinarily high earnings and endorsements he had, noteriety, as well as status. Once the glory days were over, the inflated waistline and weight in general became a major problem for many of these athletes which was a struggle they didn't have in the past.

You might think that as well-educated or at least as well-trained as these athletes were to be able to compete at such a high level, they would have learned to take better care of their bodies as they got older. When I look at pictures of many of them on the internet on websites, I'm amazed, and these are mostly men who earned millions of dollars during their careers.

I remember years ago being asked to represent a Hollywood cosmetic company because I had such a beautiful natural-looking creamy complexion. As I looked at other women, I said, "I'll never let my skin get wrinkles like that." But then fast-forward two years, and I've never been so wrong! Age happens. I didn't put on sunscreen before going into the sun, and my love of the sun and tennis prevailed, hence the wrinkles. Now I do what is necessary so the damage doesn't get worse, just as a former pro athlete should change his eating habits and exercise to prevent getting in worse shape.

I also think most former greats didn't realize how difficult it would be as they got older to maintain not just muscle tone but their weight as well. Many of them thought that because they worked out for hours and hours in their younger years, it would carry them over; but it didn't, and it won't. No matter who you are, you have to do some form of moderate exercise at the very least every other day of your life if you want to be healthy. There is no exception to this rule, famous or not. To see these former muscular men now flabby is not a pretty sight. Many may have thought because they were so famous and idolized they would be immune to illness from obesity, but that's just not the case. Some are finding out the hard way, with their physicians telling them they have to change their lifestyle for the rest of their lives if they want to live out their lives in a healthy manner, just as you and I do. And it's better to start now.

> "The first time I see a jogger smiling, I'll consider it."—Comedian Joan Rivers

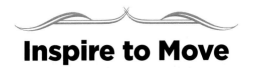

Inspire to Move

"Exercise"….bodily exertion especially for the sake of improving one's health or training.

Walk: walk the mall, walk the dog, walk in the woods, walk by the sea, just walk!

Stroll, tread, step, saunter, pace, wander, roam, stray; jump, hop, leap, lift, pull up, push up, stretch, tramp, march, ramble, traipse, trek, twist, climb; crawl, glide, slide, scrub, rub, plant, rake, swim, gym, run, zip, flip; prance, dance: bob, boogie, hoof it, hustle, jive, rhumba, samba, mambo, tango, rock, shimmy, whirl, and waltz; play ball, play tennis, play football, basketball, baseball, softball, rugby, volleyball, any kind of ball including beachball, just play but don't play cards!

If you move it no matter how, you will lose it.

Good luck, god bless, be healthy and fit.

> "The only exercise some people get is running down their friends, jumping to conclusions, sidestepping responsibility, and pushing their luck."—Author unknown

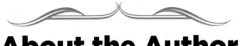

About the Author

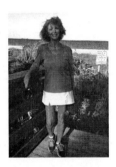

Born and raised in the Midwest, the author has spent most of her adult life in the Hawaiian Islands with a focus on fine art and physical fitness. Currently she resides in Florida with her beloved cat, "Kayla". In addition to being a weight loss coach and personal trainer, she spends her "off hours" playing tennis.